The Fundamentals

of SURGICAL

INSTRUMENTS

A practical guide to their recognition, use and care

Steve Moutrey | MSc BA(Hons) Cert. Ed RODP

tfm Publishing Limited, Castle Hill Barns, Harley, Nr Shrewsbury, SY5 6LX, UK
Tel: +44 (0)1952 510061; Fax: +44 (0)1952 510192
E-mail: info@tfmpublishing.com; Web site: www.tfmpublishing.com

Design & Typesetting:	Nikki Bramhill BSc Hons, Dip Law
First Edition:	© October 2017; reprinted September 2023
Spiral-bound	ISBN: 978-1-910079-55-3
E-book editions:	2018
ePub	ISBN: 978-1-910079-56-0
Mobi	ISBN: 978-1-910079-57-7
Web pdf	ISBN: 978-1-910079-58-4

Printed by L&C PRINTING GROUP, Tadeusza Romanowicza 11, 30-702 Kraków, Poland
Tel: +48 690 565 600; E-mail: office@lcprinting.eu; Web site: www.lcprinting.eu

Contents

Foreword

An essential component of any operative procedure is the surgical instruments that without which the surgeon could not perform his/her task. They are precision tools that have been used over the centuries and surgeons have continuously developed them to meet the increasing demands of surgical techniques and procedures. Instruments have developed from the early crude tools from bygone eras, to the intricate and precise instruments we see in modern practice and the surgical procedures of today.

Over many hundreds of years these instruments have been developed and used in many various designs, forms, sizes and shapes — each having their own specific task. Surgeons themselves have played an important role in their design and development through the ages, developing them to meet the needs for constant improvement and innovation in surgical practice. Surgeons have developed, and will continue to develop, instrument design to facilitate his or her particular needs with an understanding of the surgical task to be undertaken.

Instruments have developed from basic tools made from a variety of materials, such as ivory, bone and wood, to name but a few, to the precision instruments we now have available in the modern perioperative environment. These differing instruments range from the large to the micro, each having their own task to fulfil, whether it is to facilitate orthopaedic surgery, vascular surgery, microsurgery, ophthalmic surgery, or any other specific field of surgery.

Surgeons and surgical practitioners/assistants, as the instrument 'operators', and theatre staff, as the 'handlers' and 'maintainers', each have their own tasks to perform which demand a good understanding of the differences in how these instruments are used, what they are used for and how they are made and cared for with cognisant appreciation of the potential damage to both patient and instrument if used incorrectly. It is therefore essential that all practitioners within the perioperative environment are able to identify, use and care for the instruments within this setting and are able to both prepare and use them appropriately for all surgical cases. Misuse of instruments can place both the patient and the practitioner at risk and may become both injurious and costly if handled incorrectly and/or damaged during use.

The emphasis is incumbent upon both surgeons and theatre practitioners to gain a basic knowledge of instrumentation to allow for safe practice and surgical assistance, recognising that safety for the patient and practitioner is paramount. Good instrument care will provide a tool in practice that is sound and fit for purpose.

This book provides a basic introduction to the 'surgical instrument' in its various forms. It presents sufficient knowledge and information for those surgical personnel who use and care for instruments on a daily basis. The reader will gain a deeper understanding to allow for safe practical use. The information provided will be ideal for junior doctors, surgeons under training, scrub practitioners, nurses, operating department practitioners (both qualified and as students), surgical technologists and medical students. In addition, the book will be useful for any support workers in a theatre/surgical environment. Once the basic knowledge of surgical instrumentation has been gained, the practitioner will then be in a better position to perform their task, or assist the surgeon — providing a tool that is sound, useable and safe.

Steve Moutrey, MSc BA(Hons) Cert. Ed RODP
Senior Lecturer
School of Health Sciences and Social Work
University of Portsmouth
Portsmouth, UK

Reviews

After careful review of this text, I am impressed by Steve Moutrey's writing style, which is clear, direct, and succinct. Its audience is clearly entry-level surgical personnel, and the author understands that historical context serves as an important precursor to classification, function, care, and use of surgical instrumentation.

Mr. Moutrey's experience as a practitioner and educator is evident in his writing. As a former surgical technology educator and author of similar texts, I can attest to the difficulty of presenting entry-level surgical instrumentation. The author offers a simplified discussion enhanced with relevant illustrations that will reduce any confusion on the part of the student.

It is important to note that Mr. Moutrey has constructed his textbook to comply with the curricular requirements of the latest edition of the Association of Surgical Technologists' Core Curriculum.

Jon Paul Price, BSOE MBA
Healthcare Education Advisor/Consultant;
Former CEO, Accreditation Review Committee for
Surgical Technology and Surgical Assisting;
Former CEO, National Board for
Surgical Technology and Surgical Assisting

This text is a clearly written guide to the concept of surgical instrumentation, aimed at both pre- and post-registration students within the perioperative environment. The format is logical and gives not only factual information, but also historical context and practical advice. I envisage that this would become a standard reference for perioperative students, particularly student operating department practitioners, as well as a supportive text for perioperative staff moving between surgical specialties.

Steve Moutrey's experience as a practitioner, educator and manager is evident in the clarity of explanation and discussion of what is a potentially bewildering subject. The wealth of illustrations support the text and should prepare the reader for the practicalities of instrument identification and handling.

An essential perioperative text that fills a niche not currently addressed, I would highly recommend [the book] for all perioperative students who wish to gain a comprehensive introduction to surgical instrumentation.

Roger King, BA Cert. Ed PgCert (Res) RODP
Senior Lecturer/ODP Course Leader
University of West London, UK

Scrub practitioners and, more recently, the surgical first assistant sit at the very heart of the 'surgical team' but at present, there are simply not enough of them in the UK's NHS or indeed, elsewhere. The key, therefore, is to train as many as show a desire, willingness and aptitude for the role. However, the start of training can be a daunting time; the operating theatre staff hierarchy and environment can in themselves be intimidating and the simple volume of information and 'apprenticeship-based' workload that confronts the new trainee can, potentially, turn them off before they are ever 'turned on'! Worthy of note too, would be the importance of this book as an addition to the armamentarium of 'learning tools' for medical students and junior doctors who are about to undertake surgical practice and rotations. Rarely, if ever, do they receive any formal tuition covering this topic prior to them entering surgical practice and yet, they would be expected to assist in surgery and learn experientially 'on-the-job', quickly. Reading and revising from this text would give them a greater understanding of instrumentation prior to their 'first steps' in practice.

Steve Moutrey has a vast experience in the operating theatre environment; in an earlier military career — including active service, in field theatres, during the Falklands campaign — and more recently, embedded in both the NHS in teaching hospitals, undertaking a complete range of emergency and elective surgery, and in independent (NHS) treatment centres, with their rapid turnover of elective surgical procedures alone. Now, his experiences are being put to optimal use within a higher education setting at the University of Portsmouth; covering teaching and developmental roles in all perioperative courses and allied areas, as a Senior Lecturer within the School of Health Sciences and Social Work. The teaching commitment is primarily for operating department practice, but also involves paramedic science, nursing, radiography and speech and language therapy for specialist topics therein.

This book is aimed primarily at the scrub practitioner trainee, just starting out. It will also prove to be a useful text for other professions and learners including nurses, medical students, surgeons in training and others requiring a fundamental knowledge of surgical instrumentation. It describes in pictures and words the basic surgical instrumentation that will be found in all operating theatres throughout the NHS and similar environments, allowing easy and instant recognition of a large number, of the vast array, of instruments that surgeons and their assistants will need during any given operation. Simple explanations of why each instrument has evolved and how each is used, are given. In particular, how instruments are placed together as surgical 'sets' for given procedures will be of immense help — to provide the new trainee with a mental image of what to expect when equipment packs are first opened. The individual instrument photographs will, if the book is frequently delved into, allow instant recognition by name, but with a background understanding of function and how the particular instrument should be used to best advantage and importantly, how it should be looked after and maintained.

As an adjunct to the 'apprenticeship' of becoming a scrub practitioner — simply, an absolute key member of the modern day surgical team — this book will be a most welcome and helpful tool in itself, allowing the new trainee to gain an early understanding and confidence with surgical instrumentation and function.

Steve Barker, MB BS BSc MS FRCS
Consultant Vascular and General Surgeon
Royal South Hants Hospital, Southampton, UK

Steve Moutrey has a vast experience within the operating theatre environment spanning more than 40 years, starting his career in the Royal Navy (26 years) moving into the NHS and the private sector, and now he is firmly embedded within higher education as a Senior Lecturer at the School of Health Sciences, University of Portsmouth.

"The Fundamentals of Surgical Instruments — A practical guide to their recognition, use and care" is a book aimed at students and registered health care professionals alike who work within the operating theatre environment; in fact, all entering this field of work. Operating department practitioners, nurses, medical students and junior doctors would benefit from understanding the instrumentation within use today which will help in their confidence to handle the instruments when the time comes. The book covers various types of surgical instruments in current use and the various specialties these instruments are designed for, not only describing them and their use with pictorial evidence, but also providing a historical explanation of how the instruments developed into the instruments we know, recognise and use today. It is important to have the ability to physically recognise an instrument by its make-up, not just by its name, as names can vary slightly according to some users and manufacturers. This book not only covers the use of the instruments but also the care required to maintain them in peak condition to allow extended use. It would be impossible to cover every single instrument in use today due to instrument company innovation but this book does cover all aspects of instrument use and care. This is a much needed text as I have not found anything similar on the market that imparts this type of knowledge in a consolidated, informative single volume that would be useful to a range of practitioners and students.

It is clearly obvious that a lot of thought and effort has gone into putting this book together. Steve Moutrey has drawn upon his vast knowledge and experience both in field hospitals with the military and also from his time within the static theatre environment within the NHS and private sector. It will prove to be a valuable teaching and learning tool to all who read it, particularly the reference to the historical beginnings of the instrumentation, which is a fascinating aspect that should be understood by any user with the instruments they handle.

Terry Pugh, FAETC IOSH RODP
Theatre Clinical Manager
Queen Alexandra Hospital, Portsmouth, UK

Chapter 1

BASIC SURGICAL TECHNIQUES AND INSTRUMENT CLASSIFICATION

History

Surgery requires planned and accurate incisions using appropriate instruments to facilitate these. Historically, the visible anatomy available to a surgical practitioner was through trauma, and its understanding came from direct observation of this anatomy through these wounds. The development of surgical practice progressed through extending these traumatic wounds to gain access and vision, enabling the practitioner to facilitate such procedures as removal of foreign objects, for example, in battle trauma. It was the extension of these wounds that required the development of 'cutting' tools to seek the problem within the wound and to allow full visualisation of the internal structures. This brought about the development of relevant incising devices, or as we have come to know them now, as scalpels useful for draining of abscesses, trepanning skulls, amputations and, latterly, elective incisions for procedures such as cultural circumcision and cutting for bladder stones. These cutting tools or knives probably arose from the domestic knife, sword or cutlass that proved so adept at making an unintentional incision in the first place. The 'blade' was developed from many differing materials dependent upon the type of procedure performed; plant, mineral and animal products were used to useful effect. The lancet, a double-edged blade, was made from flint, shaped into a double-edged point to make a stab incision. Various bones and ivory were also fashioned into blades to provide incisions to denature or excise dead tissue. Shells and animal teeth, in particular, shark's teeth, were all employed to stab or cut skin and tissue. The scalpel, cutting tool or saw, therefore, was the embodiment of a surgical instrument design and its development into specific metal implements. To facilitate differing procedures, the blade has been transformed into a multi-purpose instrument, made from metal being both unserrated and serrated; the serrated for use as a saw to cut through bone as in the trephine used on the skull, and the basic hand saw to perform amputations, both requiring differing actions of use to that of the 'knife'. The sharp, single-edged blade to make accurate and clean incisions was probably derived from the blade that was folded away into a cover, as in the barber's cut-throat razor. The handle, which could have been made from tortoiseshell, protected the blade and the surgeon as he carried it. The blade was folded away inside the handle which protected the surgeon from inadvertent personal injury, whilst it also protected the actual blade from being damaged or blunted. During the early 20th century these knives gradually disappeared and became solid, fixed-bladed instruments.

Cutting instruments that were developed, alongside the saw to cut through bone, were certainly derived from the carpenter's tools of the day — these became the chisels, osteotomes and gouges we now use in modern times. These were used for dismemberment by the surgeon to remove fingers, toes and hands as they thought it provided a quicker and less painful way of amputation due to the speed with which it could be performed. These were normally by 'through-joint' amputation; using this technique, bone did not need to be cut, so facilitating a speedy procedure and consequently a less painful patient experience.

The discovery of bronze brought about the use of metal in the manufacture of instruments, providing blades and lancets for bleeding patients. Later, with the smelting of iron, further enhancing of the manufacturing process was possible. Modern surgical instruments are made of stainless steel, a combination of various metals, with the addition of carbon, to chromium and iron. This combination adds to the strength of the instruments and increases their resistance to corrosion, especially with repeated exposure to cleaning and sterilisation. The high percentage of carbon adds to their strength, making them harder — especially important for surgical blades, allowing them to remain sharper for longer. Chromium is the additive that increases resistance to corrosion. Most modern instruments have various types of finish. Highly polished finishes help to protect the instrument from corrosion and allow repeated cleaning and sterilisation; most instruments have this type of finish. The main problem with this finish is that of glare and distraction to the surgeon during use, due to reflection of bright light. A dull finish overcomes this problem as it is less reflective but it can be more susceptible to staining over repeated use. A black chromium finish to the instrument is non-reflective, eliminating all glare and is the finish of choice in microsurgery when using a microscope; also, when using lasers, it may help to prevent deflection of the laser beam from the instrument.

Some modern alternatives to metal instruments may be seen in microsurgical blades. Disposable, carbon steel blades, commonplace now, are being replaced in some practice by new materials. In ophthalmic surgery, diamond blades are being used for an ultra-sharp and precision cutting edge. Lasers are also being employed, using laser light energy to make incisions in tissues.

Hand saws are being replaced with power tools carrying disposable oscillating saw blades, which cut through bone more accurately and with a consistent sharpness. An oscillating blade also causes less tissue damage to surrounding structures and tissue. All blades and drill bits are now being provided as single use and disposable, which ensures a standard and consistent sharpness to the cutting edge.

Instruments, their manufacture and materials used in their production, will no doubt continue to be developed to meet the needs of the surgeon and his/her task. Manufacturing companies will continue to respond to these changes as surgeons continue to develop new techniques and procedures. A suitable instrument will always be required to meet these needs and developments, and the surgeon will always be in the forefront of their design to facilitate these surgical demands.

Classification

Surgeons use techniques that will require him/her to perform tasks and interventions in a coherent and rational way; to this end he will need to:

- CUT (separate or dissect).
- GRASP (hold and clamp).
- HOLD BACK (retract or push back).
- SEARCH (examine or visualise).
- REMOVE (suction or mop).
- SUTURE (approximate and return tissue to an intended anatomical norm).

Surgical instruments can be divided into a number of groups that describe their function or specific use. They may also relate to the part of the body or tissue type they are designed to be used on — this, in particular, will determine the design of a surgical instrument. It comes as no surprise that surgical instruments have various names in different hospitals or operating theatres, and there may also be no standard names for some, as many have been devised by particular surgeons for their own specific operations and uses. What is important about an instrument is the purpose it has been designed for and the type of procedure and task it has to perform.

There does, in fact, seem to be an enormous variety of instruments currently available — and this list will become more comprehensive as surgical techniques improve and develop with new procedures and operative techniques. In many surgical instrument catalogues from leading surgical suppliers, you will find a bemusing variety in the tens of thousands to choose from. What is important, therefore, is to categorise these instruments into a cohesive classification framework that you can fit each type of instrument into, allowing for recognition and the purpose of its use. It is virtually impossible to recognise every instrument, from every surgical speciality, by name, but so long as you have a basic understanding and knowledge of the instrument's distinguishing features, what it is used for and the tissue to be used on, the recognition of its name and use of the more commonly used instruments will become well known and second nature.

Distinguishing features

Instruments can be identified by their distinguishing features:

- Shape. Instruments vary in shape according to the area of the anatomy to be operated on; different shapes giving better access to otherwise inaccessible areas allowed for with basic straight instruments. Instruments can be curved or straight; the curve of the instrument may be curved on the flat, or curved on the side.
- Size. Micro (smaller) delicate instruments for use on eyes, or small nerves/vessels or standard larger instruments used on more robust and durable tissues such as muscle or tendon. Larger and heavier instruments are used on denser, stronger tissue such as bone.
- Length. Instruments of the same type or design may have many differing lengths to allow work in deeper planes of tissue, for example, long laparoscopic instruments.
- Flexibility. Rigid or malleable, as with some retractors. Some instruments are designed to pass around the shape of the structure it is being used on, for example, flexible endoscopes.
- Serrations or teeth — in or on the jaw of the instrument. These allow varying 'grips' that the surgeon needs to apply to different types of tissue. Serrations may be vertical, horizontal, crossways and these may be augmented by the instrument having teeth as well as serrations to increase the security of the hold required.

- Ratchet. A locking device, enabling the surgeon to maintain a firm, controlled grip on tissue without the need for him/her to hold on to the instrument.
- Sharp or blunt. For example, a scalpel or scissors for sharp cutting or dissection. Some instruments are designed to allow blunt dissection — these do not have any sharp cutting edges.

These instrument features are recognisable on observation and may be easily related to the job they are designed to do. The handling of these instruments and their differing design features will allow you to make informed decisions as to their purpose and use. By owning this knowledge and having an insight into the instrument's design, as the scrub practitioner or assistant, it will enable anticipation of the surgeon's needs and requirements throughout the operative procedure.

What they are used for

Dissecting forceps

Used to hold or 'grasp' tissue (■ Figure 1.1). They are spring-jawed, having no ratchet or joint, and are designed to be held between forefinger and thumb. They are probably the most commonly used instrument irrespective of the type of surgery or procedure being performed — they are found in every instrument set. Dissecting forceps come in many varieties, some with teeth, others being plain or with fine serrations for delicate tissue. They are 'fine' or 'heavy' to cope with everything from ophthalmic and vascular surgery, to the heaviest general, gynaecology and orthopaedic surgery

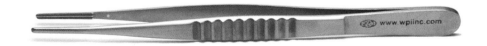

Figure 1.1. Typical dissecting forceps.

Haemostat or artery forceps

This instrument is used to 'clamp' or stop bleeding by grasping a vein or artery, for clipping off large blood vessels; hence, it is sometimes referred to as a 'clip'. A common name is the Spencer Wells forceps (■ Figure 1.2).

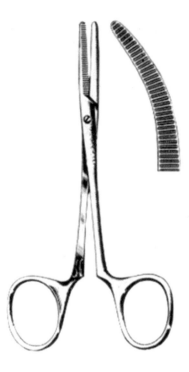

Figure 1.2. Typical artery forceps or 'clip'.

Retractor

This is used to aid the surgeon's vision of a particular structure by holding other surrounding tissue out of the way (■ Figure 1.3). They may be hand-held or self-retaining, whereby a ratchet or other mechanical device is used to hold the retractor open in a given position.

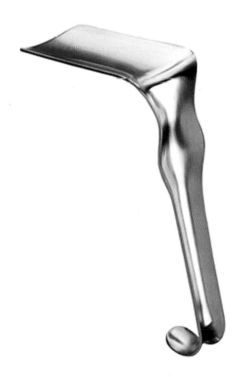

Figure 1.3. Retractor.

Scissors

Many varieties of surgical scissors are available (■ Figure 1.4), and they are used to cut and dissect tissue, cut dressings and bandages and other sundries such as sutures. They may be curved-on-flat, curved-on-side, or straight, blunt-tipped or sharp.

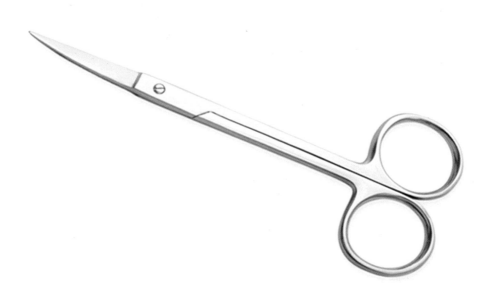

Figure 1.4. A typical pair of surgical scissors.

Scalpel

This instrument is synonymous with surgery; they have an ultra-sharp blade to make incisions in skin, and conduct fine and precise dissection, separation and parting of deeper tissues (■ Figure 1.5). All scalpels now are able to take disposable blades, and are shaped and designed for their particular surgical use and have a standard size/type number to enable its fit to a particular scalpel handle (■ Figure 1.6).

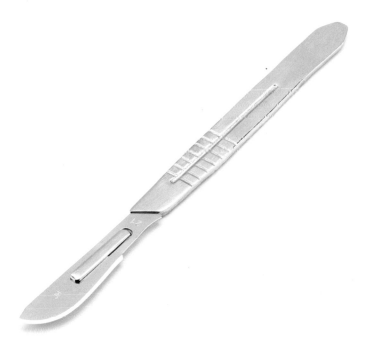

Figure 1.5. Scalpel with disposal blade attached.

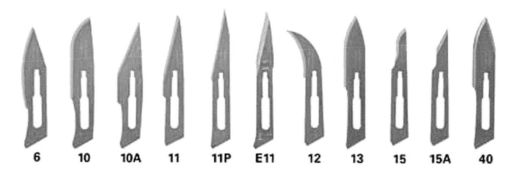

Figure 1.6. Differing types/sizes of disposable blade to fit the scalpel handle of choice.

Suction tips

When the surgeon meets differing body fluids, the obvious one being blood, they may require it to be cleared from the surgical field to allow the surgeon to have a clear view of the operative site. There are varied designs to meet specific needs — deep abdominal suctioning and surface suctioning. Also, it is an imperative instrument for suctioning in anaesthetics and airway management. The Yankauer suction tip is a common example (■ Figure 1.7).

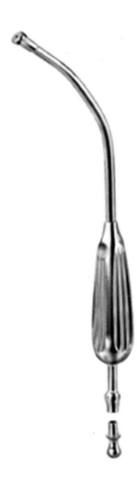

Figure 1.7. Suction cannula (tip) — (Yankauer).

Needle holders

A needle hoder is an instrument for holding a suture needle, allowing the surgeon to place or push the needle through skin or appropriate tissue to approximate the edges or planes of that tissue. A variety of designs are available, some with serrations in the jaws, others that may be plain or have teeth offering different stabilities of the needle. The needle holders in ■ Figure 1.8 show a Mayo needle holder and a needle holder which has a scissor facility built in, to cut the suture once placed and tied, using the same instrument.

a

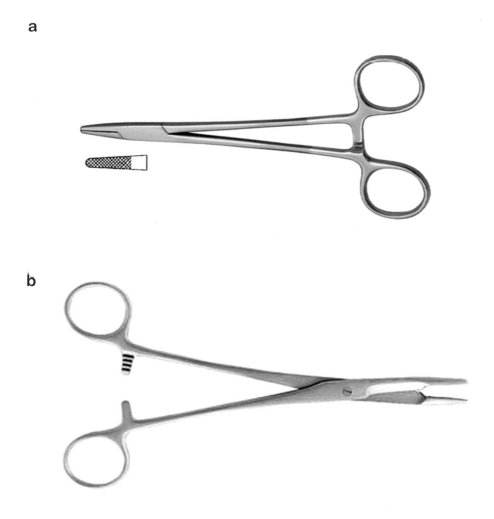

b

Figure 1.8. a) Mayo needle holder. b) Needle holder with integral scissors.

Diathermy (electrosurgical) instruments

To enable bleeding points to be sealed, or tissue to be cut/dissected, an electric current is passed through the instrument used to coagulate, or cut. These instruments are insulated, with only the active tip(s) exposed to allow only this to be applied to the relevant tissue. The insulation covering the rest of the instrument protects the surrounding tissue and structures from inadvertent burn. They may be designed as finger/thumb-type forceps (■ Figure 1.9), and are used to apply diathermy to structures at any stage of the procedure. These diathermy instruments,

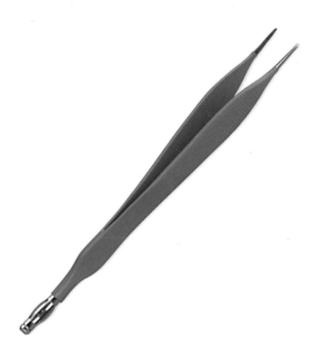

Figure 1.9. Diathermy 'thumb' forceps.

insulated with a plastic covering (preventing collateral tissue damage), come in many recognisable designs which include the various types of dissecting forceps and artery forceps as examples. Others types in use are the insulated diathermy ball tip which is used to facilitate diathermy to larger expanses of bleeding tissue beds that do not have specific bleeding points or vessels that can be 'grabbed' by forceps. The needle point and bladed point are used for incising/dissecting tissue and the pin-point application of diathermy. The single electrosurgical handle with a pencil tip (■ Figure 1.10) is an example which can be used to dissect or make incisions — arresting and cauterising bleeding points as it is used.

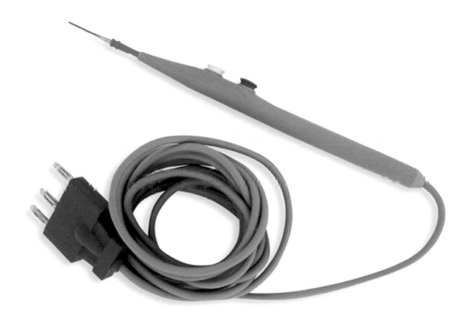

Figure 1.10. Diathermy pencil with finger switch.

Bipolar diathermy

Bipolar forceps (■ Figure 1.11) have two poles and the current passes between the instrument tips — one on both sides of the instrument, so the active and return electrode is combined within the instrument itself. Therefore, the current passes through a double-lead cable and the instrument has a 'plug' and 'socket'. The tissue is grasped between the tips which results in a more precise application of heat, minimising the transmission of heat to other surrounding tissues.

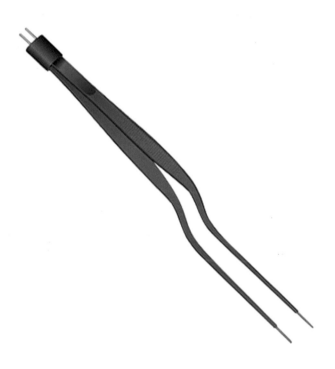

Figure 1.11. Bipolar forceps showing the double connector.

Tissue-holding forceps

These instruments are designed to grasp and hold tissue in a more definitive way. Some instruments have teeth; others that have no teeth can be applied to more friable and delicate tissue (such as bowel) without causing trauma; Babcock forceps are an example (■ Figure 1.12). Heavier, connective tissue requires a toothed instrument, as

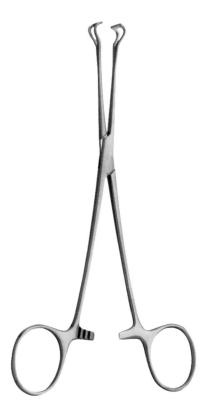

Figure 1.12. Babcock forceps.

in Lane forceps (■ Figure 1.13) to securely hold it where the 'trauma' aspect caused by the teeth is not a major consideration, but the security of the hold is, whilst tissue such as peritoneum and bowel should only be held by non-toothed instruments, avoiding perforation which would be problematic and dangerous.

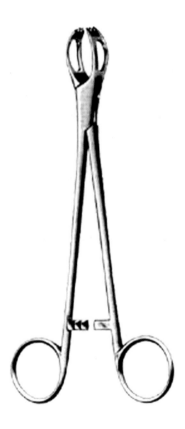

Figure 1.13. Lane forceps.

Swabs

Whilst surgical swabs are not technically instruments, it is worthy of mention here as they can and do perform a similar task to some instruments in dissection.

Obviously their primary task is to mop up body fluid and blood to keep the operative area clear, allowing full visualisation of the surgical field, so in effect they perform a role similar to suctioning.

Another good use for swabs is in aiding certain surgical techniques such as 'blunt' dissection. Some swabs are specifically designed to fulfil this role — as in 'peanut' or 'pledget' swabs (■ Figure 1.14). These are small, compact, radio-opaque swabs about 1cm in diameter which can be held in turn by a clip or artery forceps, allowing it to be used by the surgeon to separate and divide tissue from their various planes without the need to cut, or use sharp dissection. This helps maintain tissue integrity whilst opening up planes of access, and minimising tissue damage and bleeding. This type of swab is also available for laparoscopic surgery (■ Figure 1.15).

Other larger swabs (e.g.10cm x 10cm) can be wrapped around the jaws of a sponge holder and used in a similar way, used to 'push' (blunt) dissect, mop and retract deeper tissue (■ Figure 1.16). These are called 'swabs on sticks' by some and may be asked for as such.

Larger swabs or gauze packs/rolls can be used as retractors — they can be placed, for example, in the abdomen to hold back bowel from the operative area, giving the surgeon a clearer view of the site, structure, or tissue to be operated on (■ Figure 1.17). These larger swabs have a tape stitched onto them which can be clipped to the outside on the wound, onto the drapes; this aids safety by showing that a swab is being used as such and is clearly inside the abdomen, helping to identify and aid counting of the swabs. They must be removed at the conclusion of the procedure and accounted for appropriately.

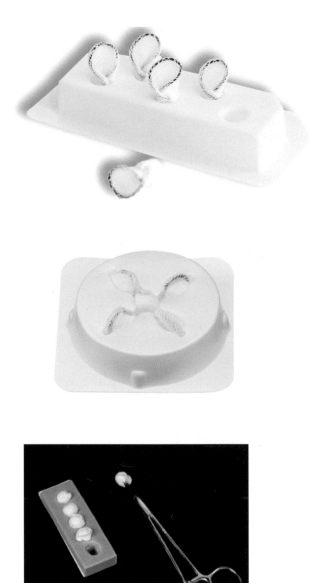

Figure 1.14. Pledgets and peanuts.

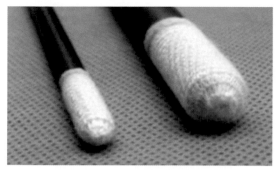

Figure 1.15. Laparoscopic peanut dissecting tips.

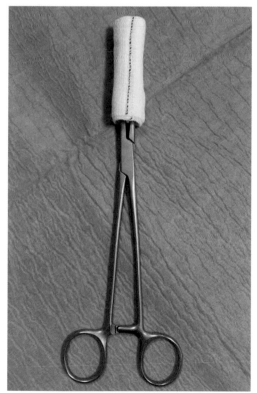

Figure 1.16. 'Swab on a stick'.

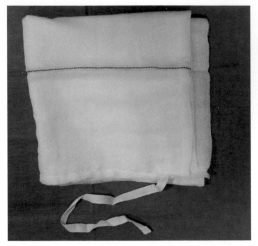

Figure 1.17. A large swab.

Chapter 2

INSTRUMENTS FOR CUTTING AND DISSECTION

Within this section it is important to discuss and expand on the group of instruments that incorporate both scissors and scalpels — the primary tools of the surgeon for cutting and incising tissue. It is also fair to say that tissue dissection does not always mean that active cutting takes place — tissue planes can be separated by the use of scissors without causing direct incised trauma. If you think of peeling an orange and taking apart the segments along the line of its natural cleavage without breaking the segment and releasing the juice — this is what the surgeon can achieve by inserting the rounded, blunt tips of the scissors, opening the jaws, thus separating the tissues in their natural planes.

Scissors

Scissors represent one of the most essential pieces of instrumentation that the surgeon requires. They provide accuracy and delicate control for every manoeuvre carried out by the surgeon. It is therefore incumbent upon the theatre staff to ensure that they are provided as well maintained, sharp and operationally sound enough to avoid both tissue tearing and 'surgeon annoyance'. The operation may well take longer as new or different scissors need to be provided to replace ones of inadequate quality — if they are available. The sharpness may be further enhanced by the inclusion of tungsten carbide inserts into the jaws to create a hardened and sharper cutting edge, allowing smoother cuts, and keeping the cutting edge sharper for longer. Most scissors have a handle with two, equal-sized ring finger loops. However, there are spring scissors (■ Figure 2.1) available, often used in microsurgery, where the handles have flat, spring-loader ends whereby the action of

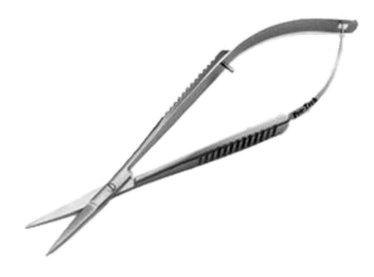

Figure 2.1. Surgical spring scissors.

cutting is achieved by pressing these handles together and where releasing the pressure allows the scissor tips to spring apart, opening the jaws.

There are many ways in which scissors can be used by the surgeon. Essential to the surgeon's armamentarium of standard instruments, they offer an indispensable tool that may be used in many ways other than just to cut tissue. The obvious way in which they are used is to cut — it is therefore important to identify the methods by which the surgeon achieves this. The direction and control of the cut made results in a desired outcome, for example, if the scissors are used with the jaws wide apart, the tissue tends to bunch up and is forced ahead of the cutting edges. Therefore, it is more advisable to utilise the instrument in such a way that the jaws are opened, showing only their tips to allow small amounts of tissue to be cut. This allows for more accuracy and stability in the action of the scissors which will cause less unwanted or undesirable tissue damage. Cutting nearer the scissor tips necessitates less closing force and greater stability when the blades are closed together.

As discussed earlier, the other main use of scissors is in blunt dissection when applied to different planes of tissue to separate tissue without causing too much damage and trauma to the surrounding structures. Using this technique, an opening is made initially, into which the tips of the closed blades can be placed to achieve separation of the tissues by gentle opening. This will result in tissue separation as the scissors are opened. Curved scissors offer superior accuracy and direction in both linear cutting and/or perpendicular cutting, allowing better visibility and control in the dissection.

A scalpel, if used, normally requires tissue to be under tension for an accurate cut; scissors can be used to cut or dissect tissue that is not under tension, therefore allowing access to areas that would otherwise prove difficult for tissue to be put under tension.

Another advantage that scissors have over a scalpel is in the technique of 'push' cutting. This is a method employed to open or cut large 'sheets' of tissue such as peritoneum or muscle fascia, pleura or pericardium. Using a knife in these areas would result in damage to their underlying structures. A small hole is made which allows the open tips of the scissors to be placed, then the scissors are 'pushed' along the tissue sheet in an accurate and controlled manor, achieving a rapid opening of the tissue plane either by blind or visible dissection along the tissue's natural fibre line.

Although there are many sizes, shapes and designs, there are basically two design types: scissors with straight blades and scissors with curved blades (curved on the flat or side). Curved bladed scissors give a greater degree of accuracy when dissecting, allowing the surgeon to make a smoother and stable cut. Cutting in deeper planes is made easier with the curved blades as better visibility can be achieved in the horizontal, downward cut. Straight scissors are better for providing a stable cut in tougher tissues due to the mechanical advantage and are usually a stronger more robust design. It is also more acceptable to use straight scissors when cutting sutures so dissecting scissors do not become blunt.

Whilst cutting sutures only the scissor tips should be used, keeping the suture, knot and sutured structure visible at all times. The knot and suture should be kept visible between the blades rather than underneath (which would happen if the blades were opened wide). A steady hand is required when cutting sutures by using either the patient or your other hand as a fulcrum to allow for greater stability and accuracy — the last thing to be avoided is to cut the suture out that has just been placed, or cut a structure which could result in inadvertent damage and disaster. Another helpful aid is to place your index finger at the hinge point of the scissors which allows for greater control and stability of the scissors when cutting.

The following illustrates a common variety of scissors encountered within surgical practice:

- Metzenbaum dissecting scissors (■ Figure 2.2).
- Mayo dissecting scissors (■ Figure 2.3).
- Stitch cutting (suture) scissors (■ Figure 2.4).
- Potts-Smith vascular scissors (■ Figure 2.5).
- Wire cutting scissors (■ Figure 2.6).
- Lister bandage scissors (■ Figure 2.7).
- McIndoe dissecting scissors (■ Figure 2.8).

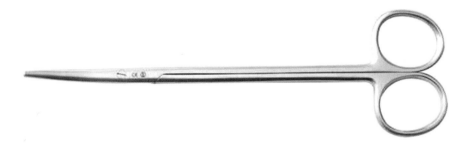

Figure 2.2. Metzenbaum dissecting scissors.

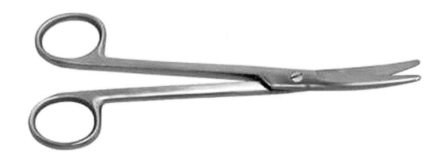

Figure 2.3. Mayo dissecting scissors.

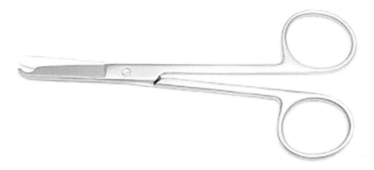

Figure 2.4. Stitch cutting (suture) scissors.

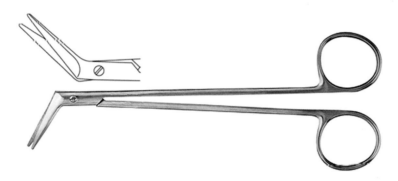

Figure 2.5. Potts-Smith vascular scissors.

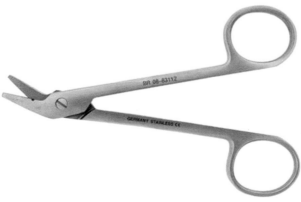

Figure 2.6. Wire cutting scissors.

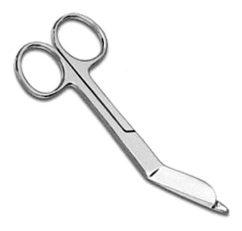

Figure 2.7. Lister bandage scissors.

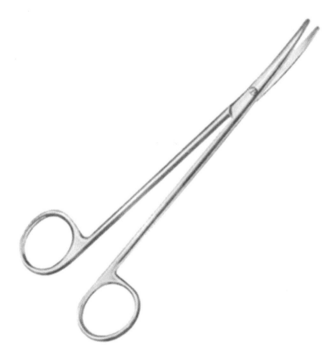

Figure 2.8. McIndoe dissecting scissors.

Scissor-like instruments

Instruments that may be classed as similar to scissors or within a group of 'cutting' instruments that are comparable, are bone cutters and bone nibblers or rongeurs. These are both similar in action and are utilised for other cutting jobs, ostensibly on heavier and tougher tissue such as bone. Because of the density and greater resistance of bone, these instruments are heavier and much more robust in their design; different types of grips and handles also allows the surgeon to achieve the desired cut due to the increased resistance from this type of tissue. Hand and palm grips/handles are employed as opposed to the finger grips or finger rings found in normal scissors. The blades or cutting ends are also designed to meet the required outcome of dissecting this denser or harder tissue. The blades are normally shorter, thicker and straight to allow the surgeon to apply the required force and to fully direct this to the tissue to be cut. Such devices can be hinged in more than one place which is a compound joint (■ Figure 2.9). These are designed to exert maximum force at the cutting tips. Conversely, the bone rongeurs (■ Figure 2.10) show a 'box' joint and heavy palm grips which are spring-loaded to aid opening once used.

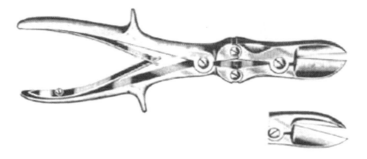

Figure 2.9. Bone cutter.

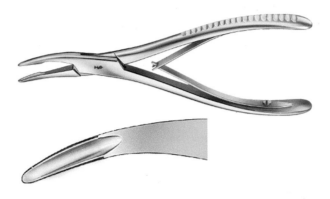

Figure 2.10. Bone nibblers (rongeurs).

Scalpels

This instrument, above all, is the most synonymous with the surgeon. Formerly, this was a solid knife (■ Figure 2.11) with an integral blade that was a reusable instrument requiring regular sharpening to keep the blade as 'keen' as possible.

After sharpening, its sharpness and edge were tested by pushing it through a thin leather skin or kid, which is leather from a young goat (most in fact were fashioned from lamb's skin as this was more readily available) stretched over a small cylindrical stainless steel tube, putting the 'skin' under tension. The best sharpness attained would be assessed by the weight of the scalpel itself being enough to push the blade through the kid. The scalpel was also assessed for any 'burrs' in the blade; if they existed, the scalpel would snag against the leather kid as it was pushed through.

With a 'scalpel in hand' the surgeon uses it for cutting through skin, fat, muscle and other tissues encountered throughout the operative procedure. Scalpels are now supplied as a separate handle that disposable, single-use only blades can be attached (■ Figure 2.12). The handles are supplied in an assortment of sizes taking

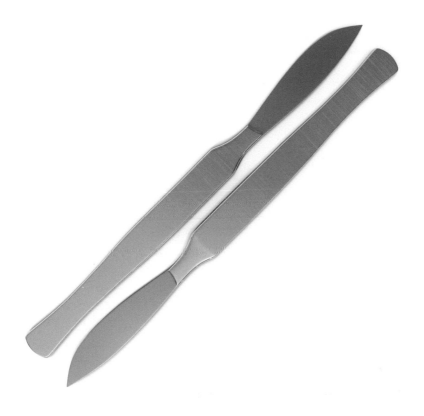

Figure 2.11. The solid knife.

these different sizes and shapes of blades which are used to facilitate a specific surgical procedure or task. Identification of the handle is achieved by its number imprinted on the scalpel handle, which correlates with the size and type of disposable blade required.

Below are the common handles and blade sizes used (■ Figure 2.12).

a

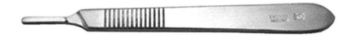

b

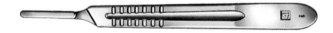

c

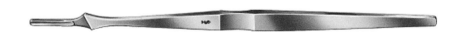

Figure 2.12. a) No. 3 handle — approximately 12cm long and will take blades of size 10, 11, 12 and 15. b) No. 4 handle — approximately 12cm long and will take blades of size 20, 21, 22, 23 and 24. c) No. 5 handle — approximately 15cm long, having a thin profile and will take blades of size 10, 11, 12 and 15.

The scalpel handle is commonly known as a "B.P. handle". This is so named after Charles Russell Bard and Morgan Parker who were founders of the Bard-Parker Company. Parker developed the single handle design in 1915 and together (Bard-Parker) they developed a method of cold sterilisation that would not dull the blades, as heat-based sterilisation tends to dull a fine sharp edge so blunting the blade.

Below is a standard range of disposable blades (■ Figure 2.13) normally seen within the operating theatre which fit the handles as described, each one having its own particular use in the surgeon's hand.

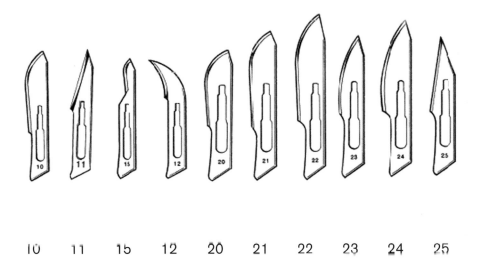

| 10 | 11 | 15 | 12 | 20 | 21 | 22 | 23 | 24 | 25 |

Figure 2.13. Disposable blade range designed to fit a scalpel handle.

Osteotomes, chisels and gouges

In this section we need to look at instruments used for cutting hard, bony tissue that are used in conjunction with bone cutters and rongeurs (described earlier). There are two main types to consider. Both present in various sizes, shapes and designs dependent upon the exact function they need to perform.

Chisel

Bone chisels (■ Figure 2.14) are seen in the dental surgical setting more than in orthopaedics; however, not exclusively. A chisel is an instrument that has been modelled on, and is similar to, a carpenter's wood chisel. It is used for cutting or cleaving bone tissue where the cutting edge is bevelled on one side only — the shank or handle may be straight or angled; the blade may also be straight or curved.

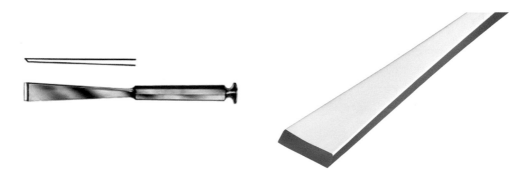

Figure 2.14. Chisel with bevel on one side of the blade only.

Osteotome

A common surgical tool in orthopaedics is the osteotome; as with the chisel, they are available in a variety of sizes and are usually handed to the surgeon with a mallet. A visual check is made of the instrument to ensure its serviceability, inspecting the cutting edges for chips or burrs to ensure sharpness and patient safety — see ■ Figure 2.15.

Osteotomes are similar to a chisel, but are bevelled on both sides of the blade. They are used today in plastic and orthopaedic surgery. In dental surgery, however, their use has been augmented and to a certain extent replaced by the use of drills and other power tools that drive cutting saw blades and drill burrs. The osteotome comes in various shapes and designs with straight and curved shafts and blades.

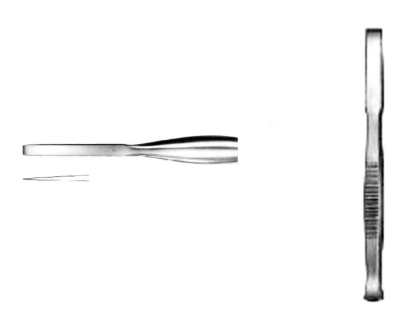

Figure 2.15. Osteotome, with a double bevel on the blade.

Gouge

A gouge, like the chisel and osteotome, is used to cut bone. It has a cutting edge similar to the chisel, but is rounded in a half-hollow shape and is used to take bone grafts and remove channels of bone utilising the rounded shape of the cutting end. Bone is cut from cancellous bone in areas such as the posterior portion of the iliac spine, just below the iliac crest. A gouge (■ Figure 2.16) is used to remove slithers of cancellous bone taken for grafting elsewhere. Various sizes and designs are provided dependent upon the type of bone required and its position.

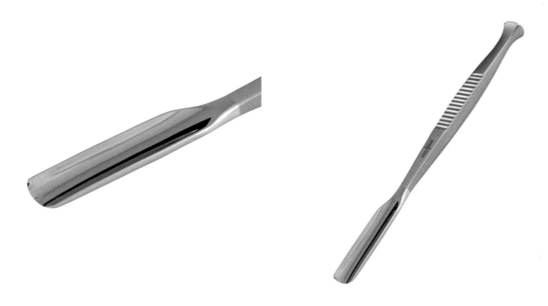

Figure 2.16. Bone gouge.

Surgical mallet

A common instrument in the orthopaedic surgeon's armamentarium, which is synonymous with this type of surgery, is the mallet. This is a heavy, stainless steel instrument and is hammer-shaped weighing between 1 and 3 pounds depending on its design and purpose (■ Figure 2.17). It is used mainly in orthopaedics but is also used by other specialties such as dental and plastics where any type of bone work is undertaken. The mallet has a stainless steel head which in some designs have a brass-filled head. Some have nylon or heavy plastic inserts which protect the smaller and more delicate instruments it is designed to strike (■ Figure 2.18). The smaller, lighter mallets are sometimes known colloquially as 'toffee hammers' as they resemble this type of hammer.

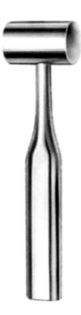

Figure 2.17. Surgical mallet.

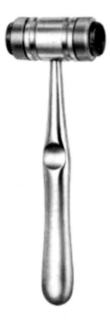

Figure 2.18. Mallet with insert.

Chapter 3

RETRACTORS AND SPECULUMS

Retractors

Instruments that are designed to expose tissue and organs within the operative site are called retractors. These instruments may be hand-held or self-retained and come in a variety of shapes and sizes. The hand-held retractors may be single- or double-ended depending upon their specific design and intended use with blades at either end (opposing ends). The simple hand-held retractor may possess a hook or blade fitted with a comfortable handle making it easier for the surgeon's assistant to hold whilst the surgeon performs his/her task. The operating ends may be sharp or blunt, depending upon the type of tissue they are designed to retract. The self-retaining retractor has mechanical means for allowing it to remain open in the wound and may be either multiply-bladed, or have two opposing blades that can be held open depending upon its use and the type of tissue it is designed to hold open; an example is the Balfour retractor (■ Figure 3.1). Many self-retaining retractors have multiple blades and in different sizes which may be interchangeable, allowing them to be used at varying depths and in different tissue types. Some self-retaining retractors can be attached directly to the operating table to give maximum stability, as in deep abdominal surgery, holding open large abdominal or thoracic wounds giving the surgeon a 'free' hand to facilitate his/her procedure through maximum exposure. Some self-retaining retractors are described as 'distractors' — these best describe the use of rib spreaders to allow the surgeon access to the thoracic cavity where the surgeon forcefully prises apart the ribs, allowing good exposure to the chest cavity.

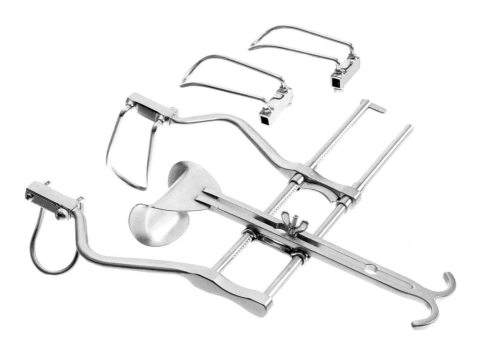

Figure 3.1. Balfour self-retaining retractor.

Below we discuss a selection of commonly used retractors — hand-held and self-retaining retractors.

Common hand-held retractors include the Volkmann retractor, the Cairns Cushing retractor, the Langenbeck retractor and the Czerny retractor (■ Figure 3.2).

Self-retaining retractors, for example, the Travers retractor (■ Figure 3.3), have a number of locking devices. The types with ring handles normally have a ratchet device (■ Figure 3.4).

Other commonly used hand-held retractors are the Deaver retractor (■ Figure 3.5) and Morris retractor (■ Figure 3.6), each of which have different sized blades. Other examples of commonly used hand-held retractors are the Richardson retractor (■ Figure 3.7), the US Army-Navy retractor (■ Figure 3.8), and the Canny-Ryall double-ended retractor (■ Figure 3.9).

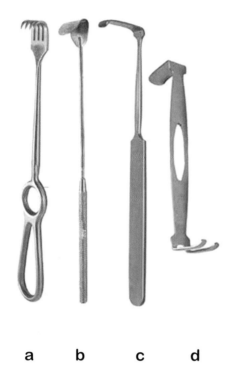

a b c d

Figure 3.2. Hand-held retractors: a) Volkmann retractor; b) Cairns Cushing retractor; c) Langenbeck retractor; d) Czerny retractor.

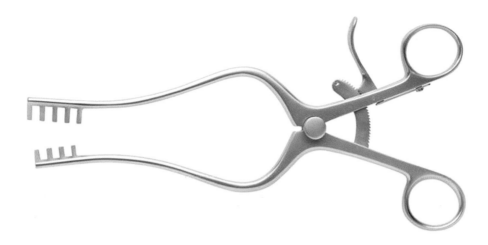

Figure 3.3. Travers self-retaining retractor.

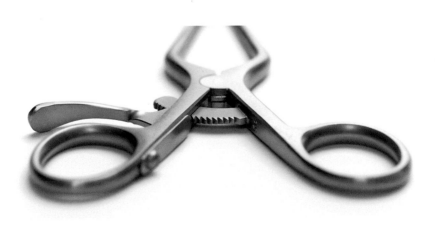

Figure 3.4. Self-retainer ratchet device.

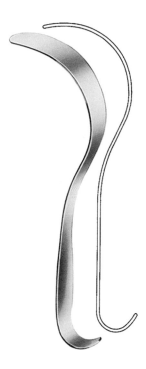

Figure 3.5. Deaver retractor.

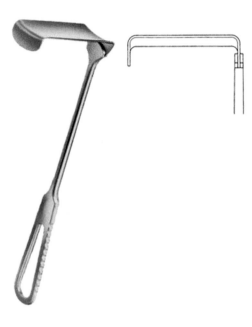

Figure 3.6. Morris retractor.

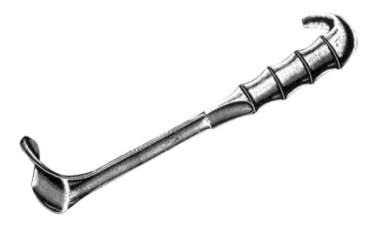

Figure 3.7. Richardson retractor.

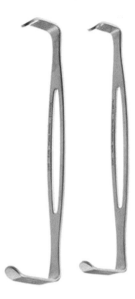

Figure 3.8. US Army-Navy retractor.

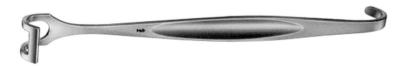

Figure 3.9. Canny-Ryall retractor.

Some self-retaining retractors have adjustable tips which aid their positioning to fit the anatomy better allowing them to 'contour' to the surface anatomy; an example is the Beckman-Weitlaner self-retaining retractor (■ Figure 3.10).

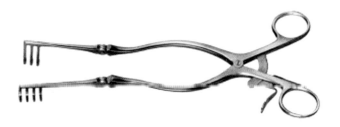

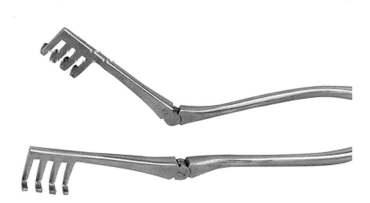

Figure 3.10. Beckman-Weitlaner self-retaining retractor showing flexible adjustable tips.

Other self-retaining retractors are designed for a specific role; an example of these is the thoracic rib spreader (■ Figure 3.11), and the larger abdominal retractors designed to fit to the operating table to ensure stability and strength of hold (■ Figure 3.12).

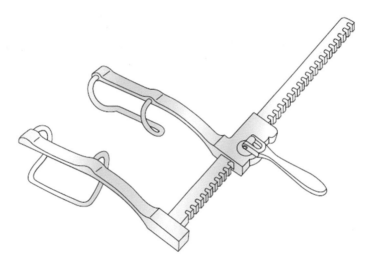

Figure 3.11. Thoracic rib spreader.

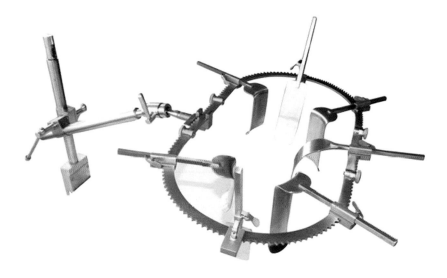

Figure 3.12. Table-mounted deep retractor.

Slings and tapes

These can be made from single-strand silicone, woven nylon, as flat tapes, or use can be made of suture material to help retract blood vessels and/or nerves.

These slings provide another form of tissue retraction for the more delicate and friable, smaller (and larger) blood vessels. They can be wrapped around a vessel which can be retracted to one side, allowing the surgeon to manoeuvre it in various directions to visualise the appropriate anatomy within a surgical site. A clip or artery forceps can be used to hold it in position, and depending on the application and the tension it is put under, it can be used to occlude the vessel as well, instead of occlusion being provided by a vascular clamp (■ Figure 3.13). Used in the same way, slings and tapes can be used to retract nerves and nerve tissue away from the surgical field, protecting them from inadvertent damage.

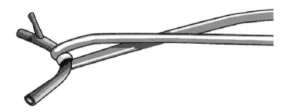

Figure 3.13. Sling around a vessel — double-wrapped which can provide occlusion.

A colour-coded system (■ Figure 3.14) may be used to determine and identify the anatomy and the different vessels being retracted or held by the slings. As these slings are potentially smaller and are not necessarily radio-opaque, careful accounting of them must take place and they must be included in all instrument, needle and swab counts to avoid inadvertent retention in a wound. Often, a single sling is cut by the surgeon — this needs to be accounted for, making sure that the instrument count remains correct.

The various slings with the colour-coding, presentation and types are shown in ■ Figure 3.14.

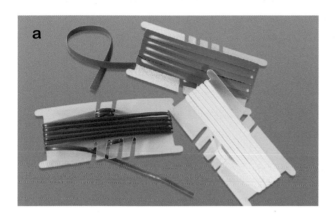

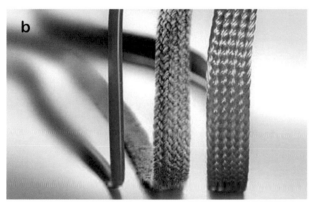

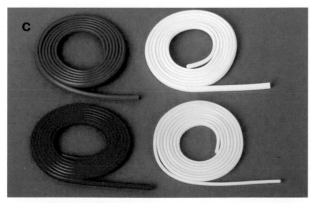

Figure 3.14. a) Silicone slings on dispensing carriers — differing lengths may be cut to size. b) Nylon tapes — various widths and colours alongside a silicone sling. c) Colour-coded silicone slings — useful for the identification of specific vessels or structures.

The lead or aluminium hand

This device is worth discussing in this section as, although not necessarily a retractor, it is used to hold a patient's hand in position with their fingers extended, allowing the surgeon access to the palm, fingers and wrist. The lead hand (■ Figure 3.15) is the most commonly used for this purpose; however, the more modern version is made from aluminium and is single use, disposable and covered in protective foam (■ Figure 3.16). The lead hand is expensive and with use over a period of time, the 'fingers' can break off requiring replacement.

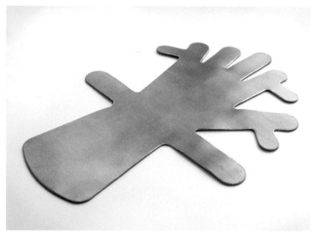

Figure 3.15. Traditional lead hand.

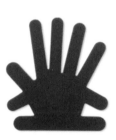
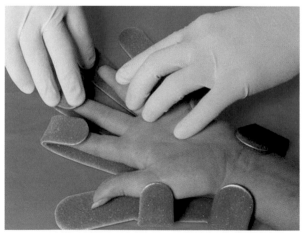

Figure 3.16. The aluminium hand showing it being positioned. This is a disposable version with foam protection.

The other advantage to using the lead hand is that the surgeon may not necessarily have suitable surgical assistance and may need to work alone with only a scrub practitioner performing a dual role scrubbing in, so they will not be able to fully commit to dedicated assistance. The lead hand, once positioned, will 'free-up' the scrub practitioner to assist as needed, without distracting him/her from their primary role in looking after the instrument trolley and count.

Other purpose-designed devices are available and can be used instead of the lead hand, such as the Vickers hand restrainer (■ Figure 3.17) — these are expensive and cumbersome. Some surgeons have devised other more readily available aids

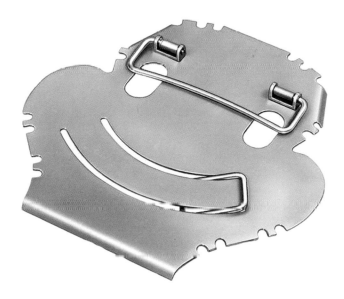

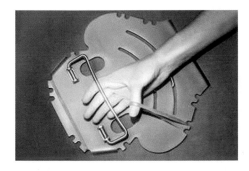

Figure 3.17. Vickers hand restrainer.

which can be obtained from ordinary domestic sources such as a basic 'cake rack' covered with a towel or gauze pad, with elastic, rubber bands to hold the fingers in position. This would provide an equally robust method of securing the hand at a fraction of the cost.

Speculums

Vaginal speculums

These are instruments that have a similar use to that of surgical retractors. They are used to allow the surgeon to gain access to tissue or structures through a body orifice, most often in gynaecological use. Their design takes the form of the orifice structure being accessed. In use, they open the orifice by 'retracting' the structures forming the orifice opening, to allow exposure and observation of tissue within that orifice, which is why they have been included within this section as they perform a specific retraction function.

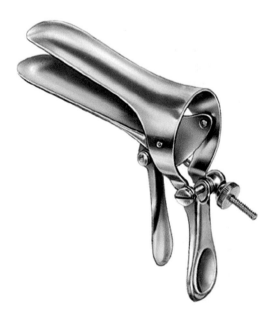

Figure 3.18. Cusco vaginal speculum.

These speculums can be used to expose areas such as the vagina, anal canal, nasal passages and ear canal (external auditory meatus).

Probably one of the best known is the Cusco vaginal speculum (■ Figure 3.18), which is a two-bladed instrument that can be opened on its hinge once inserted to view the vagina and cervix. Once inserted, it can be held open by a screw device or ratchet on the handle making it a self-retaining speculum — holding the blades open *in situ*.

Some vaginal speculums are designed specifically for a surgical function and to be used intra-operatively; the most common are the Sims and Auvard speculums.

The Sims speculum (■ Figure 3.19) is a double-bladed, hand-held speculum, also used to visualise the vagina and cervix. Depending on the patient position in lithotomy and how far the patient is positioned down the table, it can be held in place or placed so it holds itself *in situ* with the lower blade tucked into the perineum. When positioned, it retracts the posterior wall of the vagina.

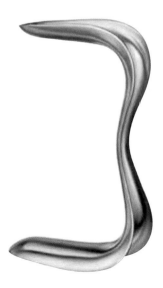

Figure 3.19. Sims vaginal speculum.

The Auvard vaginal speculum (■ Figure 3.20) is a more specialised operative instrument with a single blade attached to a half-tubed channel positioned at about 90° to the blade. At the base of the channel is a weight, which allows it to hang in place once inserted to open the vagina and retract the posterior wall. This weighted speculum is used operatively with the patient in the lithotomy position for all vaginal surgery and allows the surgeon a free hand whilst operating.

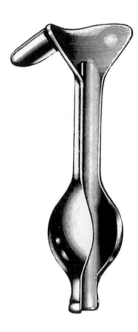

Figure 3.20. Auvard speculum.

Rectal speculums

For rectal surgery, a number of speculums exist from cylindrical tubes to speculums with multiple blades. A proctoscope (■ Figure 3.21) allows visualisation of the anal canal and the sigmoidoscope (■ Figure 3.22), which is much longer, allows visualisation of the rectum and lower sigmoid colon. Both are ridged metal or plastic tubed speculums that may have a light source attachment, especially the sigmoidoscope. These speculums have a blunt trocar-like device or obturator, with a rounded end to allow insertion via the anus without causing trauma and then removed to facilitate visualisation once inserted. To aid visualisation of the rectum and lower sigmoid colon, an inflating balloon device is usually attached to the sigmoidoscope so it can be inflated once inserted.

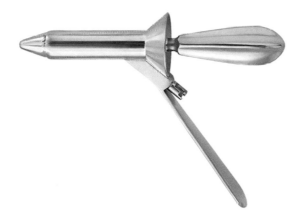

Figure 3.21. Proctoscope.

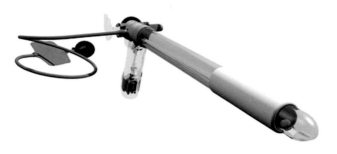

Figure 3.22. Sigmoidoscope with an inflation balloon.

The non-cylindrical or tube type of speculum has blades that can be opened once inserted into the rectum to allow full visualisation and procedures to be carried out, as in haemorrhoidectomy or haemorrhoid banding. Once opened, using the handle, the self-retaining properties of the speculum allow the surgeon a hands-free approach to the procedure. Two examples of these instruments are the Parks speculum (■ Figure 3.23), which may be used with two or three blades and the Eisenhammer speculum (■ Figure 3.24), which has a thumbscrew device to keep the blades open once inserted.

Nasal speculums

Nasal speculums are designed with smaller and flatter blades to open the nostrils and advance into the nasal passages. These, like other speculums, can have a handle which opens when squeezed together and be retained in the open position, or just held open using finger and thumb utilising a spring handle. This speculum is the Thudichum nasal speculum (■ Figure 3.25) and is probably the most common one in nasal use to visualise the anterior aspect of the nasal septum, nares and anterior/posterior/middle turbinates.

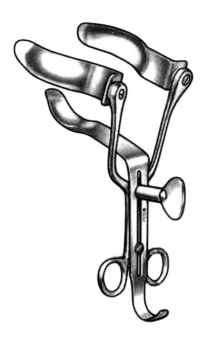

Figure 3.23. Parks rectal speculum.

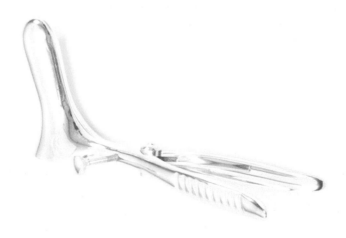

Figure 3.24. Eisenhammer (Pratt) rectal speculum.

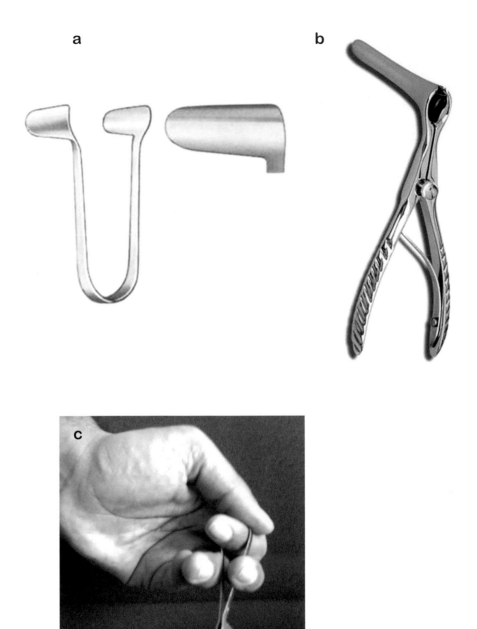

Figure 3.25. a) and b) Thudichum nasal speculums. c) Showing the finger and thumb placement when using the Thudichum spring-handled nasal speculum.

Aural speculums

For examination of the ear, an aural speculum is used (■ Figure 3.26). These are used diagnostically and can be fitted to an auroscope which can be both battery and/or mains powered, or used in surgery when accessing the external auditory meatus to visualise the tympanic membrane through a microscope. They are funnel-shaped and normally the operating speculum has a slot cut down the side of it allowing easier instrument manipulation and access during surgery. Some speculums are bivalved and have a hold-open device with a small thumbscrew to open the speculum blades, enabling the speculum to open up the external auditory meatus, holding it in place without having to hold it in place manually. All aural speculums come in various sizes to cope with varying external meatus diameters and sizes.

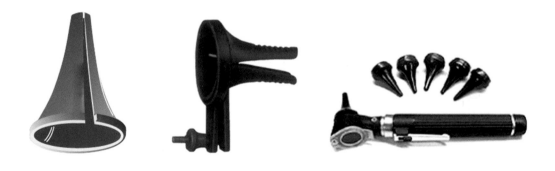

Figure 3.26. Auroscope and operating aural speculums.

Ophthalmic speculums

For surgery and examination of the eye, the eyelids are required to be held open allowing full access to the surgeon. This is facilitated using two main types: these are wire and rigid speculums. They operate in much the same way as a self-retaining retractor but are classed as a speculum. The Barraquer wire speculum (■ Figure 3.27) is probably the most widely used for modern cataract surgery, especially phacoemulsification. The wire, being spring-loaded, opens without undue stress or over-extension of the eyelids. The common rigid speculums are the Lang or Castroviejo speculum (■ Figure 3.28) and these have a self-retaining device — usually a screw fixing, to hold open the speculum blades. Both paediatric and adult speculums are available.

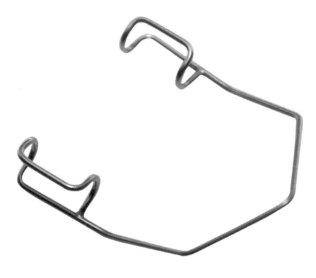

Figure 3.27. Barraquer wire speculum.

a

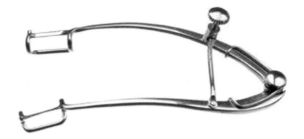

b

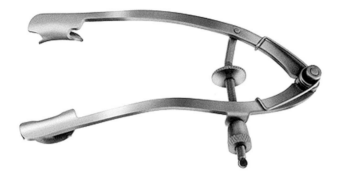

Figure 3.28. a) Lang and b) Castroviejo rigid eye speculums.

Chapter 4

FORCEPS

These are the grasping or holding instruments designed to allow the surgeon to manipulate tissue, to facilitate dissection or suturing by holding the edges of tissue or skin whilst another surgical step takes place. An example of this would be holding and perhaps turning the skin edge (■ Figure 4.1) as the surgeon approximates them together whilst placing sutures.

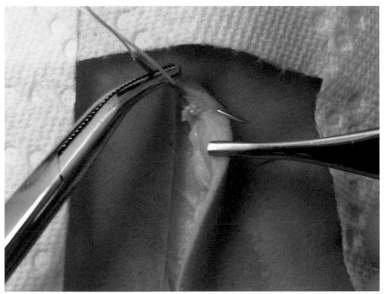

Figure 4.1. Forceps being used to grasp and evert skin prior to approximation with a suture, in this case a continuous subcuticular suture closure.

In their various forms and designs, these instruments are probably the most commonly used instrument, and are found in every instrument set, irrespective of the type of surgery being performed. They have multiple uses other than holding skin when suturing: extracting needles, passing ligatures to other instruments around vessels for tying them off, grasping vessels to apply diathermy, packing swabs and haemostatic sponges into wounds and clearing blood and clots with or without swabs and, thus, they are a versatile instrument.

These forceps are normally designed without a ratchet or locking device. They are 'pick-ups' or 'thumb' forceps and are constructed with a flattened handle that will spring back open when the hold is released. They are usually held in the non-dominant hand to grasp tissue when suturing and dissecting; they may have teeth and serrations or be smooth at the active end, and they vary in length depending upon the job they are being used for and the depth of the structure being operated on. The forceps are held so that one blade of the instrument functions as an extension of the thumb and the other blade as an extension of the opposite fingers — ■ Figure 4.2 demonstrates the forceps hold.

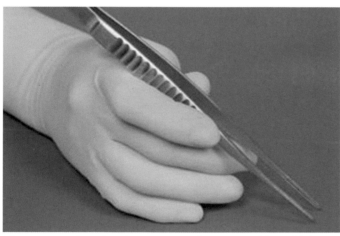

Figure 4.2. Showing how tissue dissection (thumb) forceps are used and how they are held.

The size of the forceps will also be varied, from the micro forceps used with an operating microscope, as in ophthalmics, to the large, heavy forceps used in gynaecology or orthopaedics, designed to hold heavy fibrous tissue.

Common examples are:

- McIndoe (■ Figure 4.3).
- DeBakey (■ Figure 4.4).
- Gillies (■ Figure 4.5).
- Adson (■ Figure 4.6).
- Bonney (■ Figure 4.7).
- Officer pattern (■ Figure 4.8).

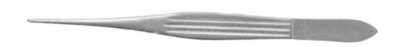

Figure 4.3. McIndoe forceps.

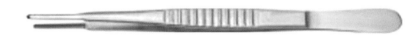

Figure 4.4. DeBakey forceps.

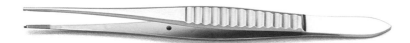

Figure 4.5. Gillies toothed forceps.

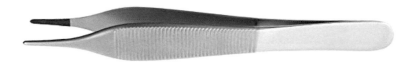

Figure 4.6. Adson forceps.

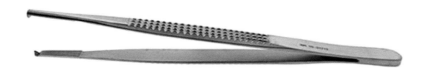

Figure 4.7. Bonney forceps.

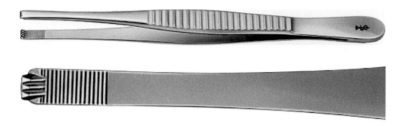

Figure 4.8. Officer pattern forceps.

In summary, forceps are used to hold, retract, stabilize, extract, pack swabs and dressings into wounds and pass ligatures. They can be used to secure and stabilize tissue on the suture needle during its extraction from the wound or tissue, or grasp the suture needle for extraction once passed through the tissue or skin.

Chapter 5

CLAMPS AND CLIPS

Clamping instruments are designed to occlude or constrict tissue, structures and vessels. They are constructed with opposing ring handles for finger control and locking ratchets aligned with or just below the ringed handles — this locks the instrument, once applied to the appropriate tissue. Arising from the ringed handles are normally two shanks leading to the working end and a box joint hinge which controls the opposing jaws of the instrument. These instruments, as described earlier, may be curved on flat, curved on the side or straight and have either blunted, rounded ends, or have sharp points. Recognition of use will come from the serrations in the jaws and these may be horizontal, vertical or cross-hatched, giving better traction and hold on the relevant tissue. Some clamps are specifically designed for holding more delicate tissue that the surgeon will not want to damage, as in vascular or gastrointestinal surgery, whilst others are used to 'crush' tissue as in some bowel resection surgery, the design of the jaws dictating their use. Some have long, flexible jaws that are constructed to prevent tissue damage when applied, as this allows for better protection of the structure being clamped. Intestinal clamps have long flexible 'non-crushing' jaws to facilitate proper occlusion as well as protecting the bowel being clamped. Some clamps have the facility to have silicone, plastic or cloth inserts, or 'boots' to cover the jaws (■ Figure 5.1), which provides extra protection when applied. They may be colour-coded if applied to hold sutures, ligatures or tapes that hold specific vessels or structures to aid identification. Clamps that have material or cloth covers are normally used for providing extra protection when clamping blood vessels or bowel.

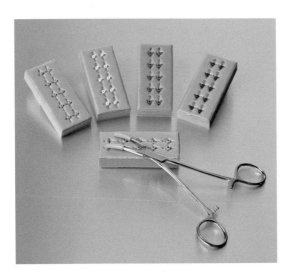 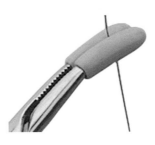

Figure 5.1. Instrument boots being applied.

Haemostatic clamps or 'clips'

Haemostatic clamps are used (normally curved on flat jaws) to occlude bleeding vessels prior to ligating or tying off these bleeders, providing haemostasis. They may also have straight jaws, these being used for various 'clipping' and 'clamping' procedures but also frequently used to clip or tag sutures and the tails on large swabs to the outside of the drapes, when swabs are placed inside an abdomen. Artery forceps may also be utilised for blunt dissection. Clamps are best used for blunt dissection where vessels occur to identify and expose them, as sharp dissection with scissors may inadvertently damage them. Commonly used examples of haemostats or artery forceps are Spencer Wells, Rochester, Dunhill and Kelly forceps.

Haemostatic forceps can clamp blood vessels which can be secured by either two clamping techniques, using the tips or the whole jaw of the instrument. With 'tip' clamping, the curved tip points towards and grasps the open vessel and includes minimal surrounding tissue. Jaw clamping allows the surgeon to grasp a large portion of tissue, normally with the tip pointing away, to allow for a ligature to be passed around this tissue and tied. They are also used in pairs to clamp uncut tissue pedicles prior to their division and ligation, for example, when dividing the mesentery at bowel resection. Since, in some instances, clamps can be used to hold tissue, they can be an effective retractor, useful in manoeuvring a mass to allow dissection around it or moving layers of tissue to gain full visualisation of the area.

Most clamps possess ring handles and a ratchet (■ Figure 5.2) for a locking device to hold the tissue securely. The anatomy of the typical clamp (■ Figure 5.3)

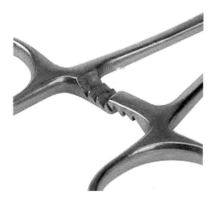

Figure 5.2. Locking ratchet.

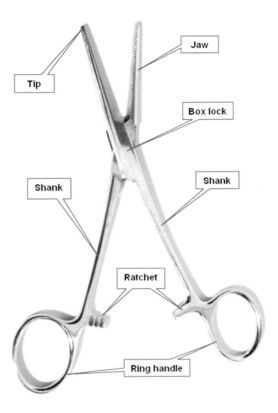

Figure 5.3. Common features of a typical clamp.

and artery forceps (■ Figure 5.4) are shown above and below. (For needle holders refer to Chapter 1.) There are variations but the common features remain the same.

The following illustrations show a range of haemostatic clamps or 'clips' that are found in common surgical practice:

- Kelly artery forceps (■ Figure 5.4).
- Spencer Wells artery forceps (■ Figure 5.5).

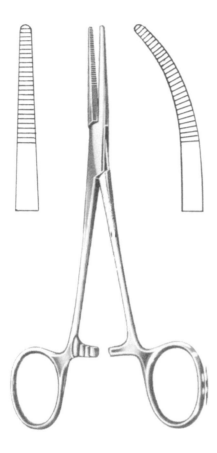

Figure 5.4. Kelly artery forceps.

- Dunhill artery forceps (■ Figure 5.6).
- Rochester (Pean) artery forceps (■ Figure 5.7).
- Kocher (Ochsner) toothed artery forceps (■ Figure 5.8).
- Mosquito artery forceps (■ Figure 5.9).

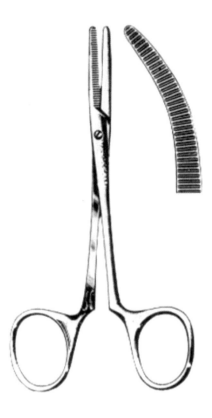

Figure 5.5. Spencer Wells artery forceps.

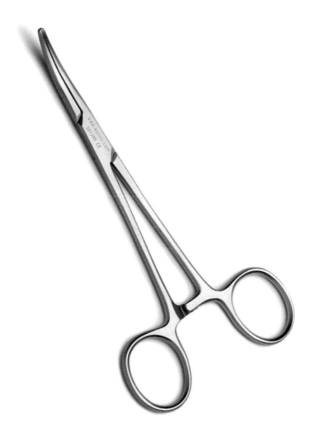

Figure 5.6. Dunhill artery forceps.

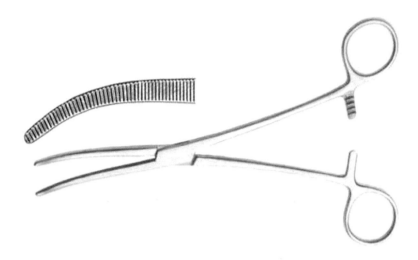

Figure 5.7. Rochester (Pean) artery forceps.

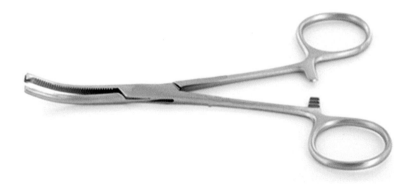

Figure 5.8. Kocher (Ochsner) arterial clamp, showing toothed tips.

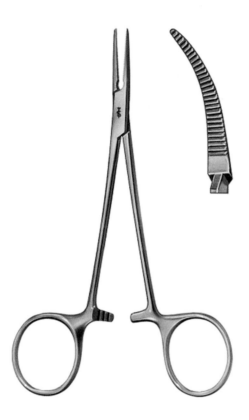

Figure 5.9. Mosquito forceps.

Two types of forceps that may be used for similar procedures are the Mixter (■ Figure 5.10) and Lahey right-angled forceps (■ Figure 5.11). They are commonly used in a number of specialised situations — working in obscured surgical sites to clamp and dissect vessels, tubular ducts and structures. They come in a variety of sizes and lengths. Lahey forceps are commonly used for cholecystectomy, for applying to and grasping the cystic duct and/or common bile duct. They are also used for dissecting and grasping arteries and veins in vascular surgery. Lahey forceps have longitudinal serrations, whereas the Mixter forceps have full-length horizontal serrations.

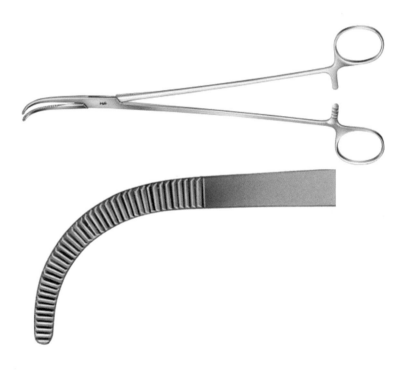

Figure 5.10. Mixter forceps showing the tips.

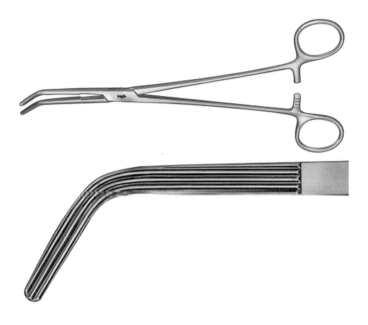

Figure 5.11. Lahey forceps showing the right-angled tip.

Vascular clamps

These are instruments that are used during surgery on arteries and veins. They are designed to stem the blood flow into and from areas that are being operated on, and to stem blood flow from ruptured vessels. They are manufactured in a variety of shapes and sizes to meet the needs of the procedure being performed and can be used in various areas, for example, to stem blood flow to the brain, which may require temporary clamping of the carotid artery, or for clamping the abdominal aorta for the repair of an abdominal aortic aneurysm (AAA). Vascular clamps can be used in surgery on all vessels encountered and include: angled, straight, curved aortic (■ Figure 5.12), Satinsky (■ Figure 5.13), bulldog (■ Figure 5.14), DeBakey (■ Figure 5.15) or Fogarty (■ Figure 5.16) clamps, and are useful for removal of organs, anastomosis of arteries and in transplant surgery. The clamps usually have a micro- or

79

non-serrated jaw (■ Figure 5.17) which run the full length of the instrument's jaw, preventing damage to the blood vessel being clamped and held. Clamps may also have silicone, foam or rubber sleeves placed onto the jaws (■ Figure 5.18) which also help to prevent damage to the vessel. It is worthy of note that these clamps are applied cautiously and slowly and not fastened too tightly; this also prevents further damage to the vessel, especially arteries. The names are suggestive of the designer/surgeon who developed them and certainly with vascular clamps, there may be a number of sizes and shapes attributed to the surgeon's name. Examples are the many varieties of DeBakey clamps available, such as the DeBakey general vascular clamp (■ Figure 5.19) and the DeBakey 'sidewinder' aortic clamp (■ Figure 5.20).

Examples of the various vascular clamps are shown in the figures below.

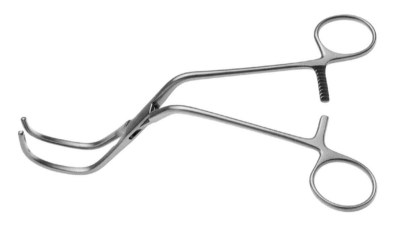

Figure 5.12. Aortic clamp.

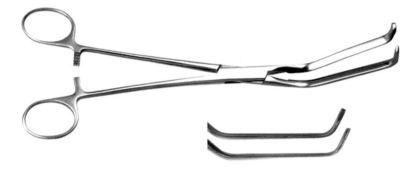

Figure 5.13. Satinsky vascular clamp.

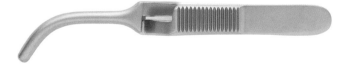

Figure 5.14. DeBakey bulldog clamp.

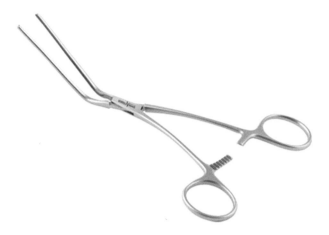

Figure 5.15. DeBakey vascular clamp.

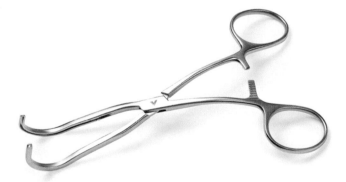

Figure 5.16. Fogarty clamp.

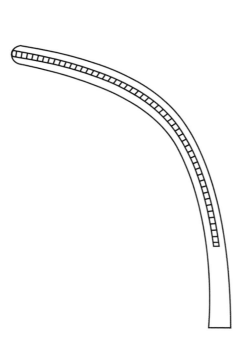

Figure 5.17. Vascular clamp jaw showing micro-serrated jaws.

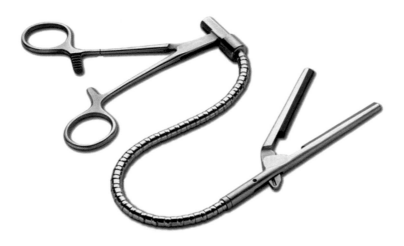

Figure 5.18. Vascular clamp with insert.

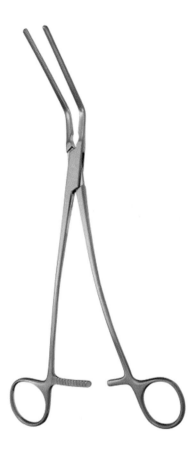

Figure 5.19. DeBakey general vascular clamp.

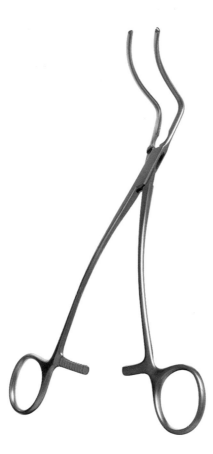

Figure 5.20. DeBakey 'sidewinder' aortic clamp.

As well as using these clamps for anastomoses, resections and in transplant surgery, they are also commonly used in neurosurgery and cardiac procedures. Surgeons need to make quick, rapid decisions during these procedures to obviously prevent a patient from bleeding out. This is more evident during emergency procedures when arteries are haemorrhaging at varied rates — from a full rupture to a slow leak. Organs need to maintain their perfusion from an arterial flow, so it becomes vital that the surgeon's decision is responded to by the correct provision of the instrument designed to meet the specific need.

Surgery of this type and nature obviously has an associated risk where vascular clamping is involved, so it becomes vitally important that the whole surgical team has an understanding of the procedure and instrumentation, to prevent delays or avoidable complications. This includes the surgical assistant, who may be required to close or release a clamp slowly, to the scrubbed practitioner who needs to anticipate the needs of the surgeon. The importance, therefore, of understanding and having a knowledge of these instruments and procedures can save lives.

Chapter 6

SUCTION DEVICES

These are devices that when attached to a vacuum source via appropriate suction tubing, are used to remove blood and body fluids, allowing the surgeon to adequately visualise the surgical field.

They have various designs and 'tips' attached to a form of handle to allow suctioning of everything from small wounds to large abdominal wounds. For larger incisions where an increased blood loss or large amount of fluid is anticipated, for example, in a hydrocoele repair, a wider bore and suction tip with multiple holes can be used — as in the Yankauer sucker (■ Figure 6.1), or for abdominal surgery a

a

b

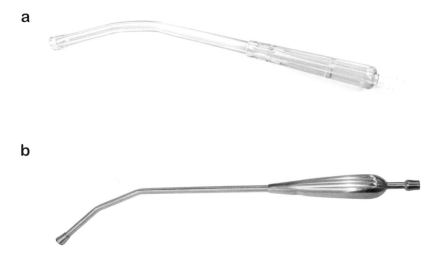

Figure 6.1. Yankauer sucker (suction tip): a) disposable; and b) metal reusable.

Poole (■ Figure 6.2) or Simpson-Smith suction device (■ Figure 6.3) may be considered.

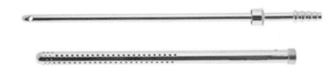

Figure 6.2. Poole suction tip.

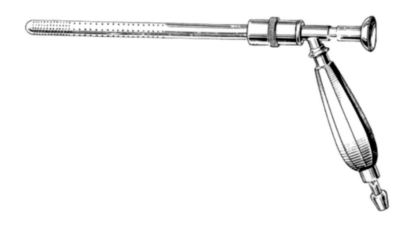

Figure 6.3. Simpson-Smith suction tip.

A suction tip with multiple holes avoids an aspiration injury where more delicate tissues may be inadvertently sucked into the tip, as in abdominal surgery where there is a danger of suctioning bowel into the sucker tip. If this occurs then either release the suction by taking the finger off the control port (for suckers that have this facility) or bend or occlude the suction tubing, then gently prise the tissue away from the sucker tip. Tissue that has become trapped in the suction tip/holes should never be forcefully pulled out; gently remove the tissue when active suction has been turned off.

Good visualisation of the surgical area to be suctioned is paramount to provide a good field of vision for the surgeon and to avoid trauma. Tissue trauma can occur if overzealous use is employed when suctioning, especially if a fine-tipped device is used, as this could penetrate or tear friable tissue causing both damage and even more bleeding.

Some suction devices, such as the Frazier suction cannula (■ Figure 6.4), have small removable tips (as in ENT procedures), and these need to be accounted for

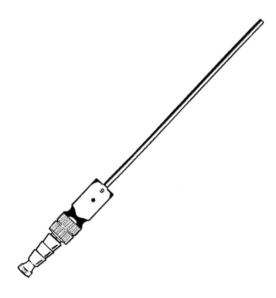

Figure 6.4. Frazier sucker showing the finger control port (fine tip).

carefully and counted with the instruments and swabs, as it is easy to lose one of them. It is also possible that the surgeon may find it necessary to unscrew or remove a sheath or tip; this must be taken by the scrub practitioner and again accounted for appropriately.

The Frazier suction tube is thinner than other suckers and is used for removing fluid from smaller and more confined spaces such as the nasal cavity or, if used with fine tips, the ear canal. It can also be employed in cranial or spinal surgery. It normally comes with a fine wire stylet which can be used to remove any tissue that blocks the lumen of the suction tube. The suction is controlled by the finger port in the handle.

A specially designed suction (irrigation) device is used for laparoscopic surgery where the surgeon needs precise suctioning with irrigation (■ Figure 6.5). The irrigation is combined within a single instrument with the suction facility, where both the suctioning is used for evacuating body fluid and blood, and the irrigation can be

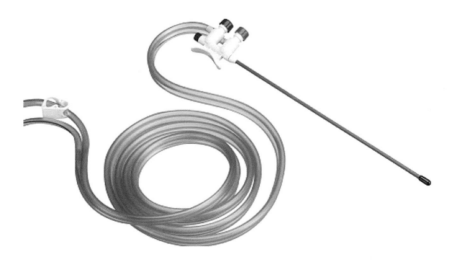

Figure 6.5. Laparoscopic suction/irrigation system.

employed using the dual control at the surgeon's finger tips. Irrigation is deployed to aid the visualisation of tissues and structures being operated on, for example, to irrigate an area that is bleeding. In this instance, the surgeon needs to identify the bleeding point so that he can facilitate suitable haemostasis; by streaming the irrigation fluid over this area, he can see exactly where the bleeding point is — suction is then applied to remove the irrigation fluid. Another prime use is to irrigate and suction bile from the gallbladder bed in a laparoscopic cholecystectomy if it becomes perforated.

The control of laparoscopic suction/irrigation is in the hands of the operating surgeon (■ Figure 6.6). Both controls can be operated single-handed, alternating between suction and irrigation as required.

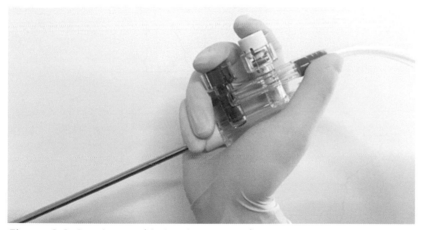

Figure 6.6. Suction and irrigation controls.

The tip of this device (■ Figure 6.7), designed in a similar way to the abdominal suction tip catheter (Simpson-Smith and Poole suction device), has multiple holes to prevent the inadvertent 'sucking' in of surrounding tissue.

Many suction tips are now provided as disposable single-use devices (■ Figure 6.8), as the reusable suction tips have cleaning and sterilising issues due to the fine, narrow bore on some — such as the Frazier suction tip. These need to be carefully cleaned with either a specially provided lumen brush (■ Figure 6.9) and/or processed through an ultrasonic cleaning bath.

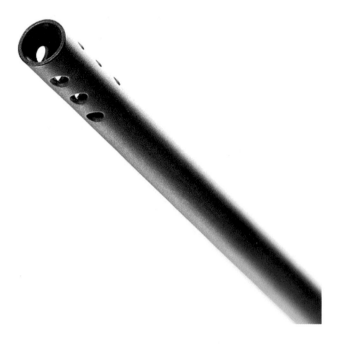

Figure 6.7. Suction tip on a laparoscopic device.

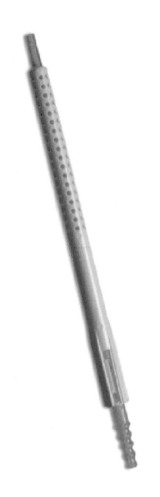

Figure 6.8. Disposable Poole sucker.

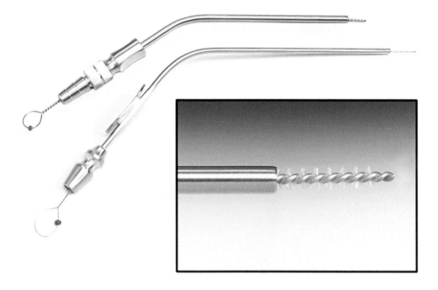

Figure 6.9. Frazier suction tip showing the lumen brush.

Chapter 7

SEARCHING AND DIAGNOSTIC INSTRUMENTS

There will be times when the surgeon cannot see or feel specific structures and will need to seek out areas within these structures. It will be important for him/her to access, examine or perform a procedure within these areas without disrupting surrounding tissue that would otherwise be inaccessible without causing excessive trauma.

To allow access to these parts there are many options open to the surgeon:

- Non-invasive techniques.
- Minimally invasive techniques.
- Surgically invasive techniques.

Many non-invasive techniques using both radiological approaches and non-radiological approaches are available to the surgeon to aid diagnosis, such as ultrasound scans, angiograms, echocardiograms and special scans such as computed tomography (CT) and magnetic resonance imaging (MRI).

Minimally invasive techniques can be accomplished by using instrumentation such as endoscopes. These can be either rigid or flexible. The endoscope is a generic name given to all instruments that are used to examine a structure or internal organ through a natural, surgically manufactured opening or orifice. Most areas of the body are available to the 'surgeon's eye' by using an endoscope through these approaches. Some of these instruments can be used intra-operatively such as the choledochoscope (■ Figure 7.1), which can be used to access and see inside the biliary system to look for blockages, i.e. stones.

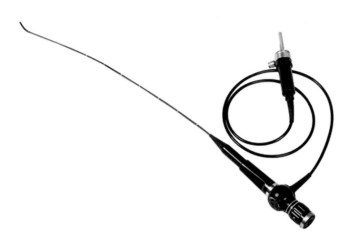

Figure 7.1. Choledochoscope.

Endoscopy is developing into a highly technical specialty that requires a range of external 'high-tec' equipment, such as stack systems containing an optical camera, processor, insufflator, light source and in many cases a compatible printing device. There is also consideration made for the provision of specialised suction/irrigation systems. These are mainly for laparoscopic procedures but are also required by surgeons utilising other endoscopes — both rigid and flexible — for procedures such as, for example, cystoscopy in urology and hysteroscopy in gynaecology. Also, other specialties such as orthopaedics use an endoscopic approach for some of their procedures, such as with arthroscopies — looking into joints. ENT surgeons also use these systems for endoscopic procedures such as sinus surgery. For most types of endoscopic surgery, practitioners need to be familiar with the tasks and normal operating functions of this equipment, from which an understanding of the problems and troubleshooting of the equipment will develop. Other instrument considerations that need to be addressed are the operative cannulas and ports that are required to facilitate placement of the endoscopic instruments used for the procedure — this will be covered later under laparoscopic instrumentation (see Chapter 11).

Surgically invasive techniques employ the use of instruments such as probes, for example, a sinus probe that has a number of differing sizes and shapes to enable the surgeon to follow a sinus tract; an example of this is the Lockhart-Mummery fistula probe (■ Figure 7.2). These are just as important to the armamentarium of the surgeon and are used to search out sinuses, unnatural tracts and cavities for blockages, stones and foreign bodies.

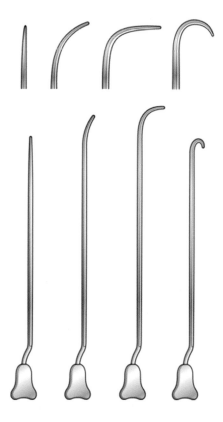

Figure 7.2. Lockhart-Mummery fistula probes.

Other instruments can be employed to remove these blockages, caused by, for example, stones. Depending upon the cause, these instruments may be handled, grasping-type forceps, such as the Randall stone forceps/graspers (■ Figure 7.3) or catheters with an inner device that can be opened within a structure to grasp/remove blockages caused by stones or blood clots, for example, a Dormia basket (■ Figure 7.4).

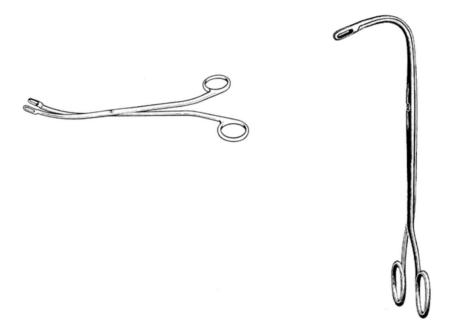

Figure 7.3. Randall stone-removing forceps.

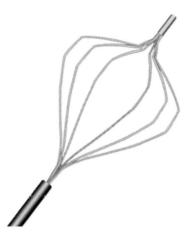

Figure 7.4. Dormia basket showing the 'basket' open ready to capture a stone.

Probing, which may be followed by irrigation, is a procedure used to assess the anatomy and function of a duct, for example, the lacrimal drainage system with the eye. It may be carried out to treat a blockage or obstruction within the lacrimal duct which may be due to stenosis from repeat chronic infection, trauma or from a congenital nasolacrimal duct obstruction. By probing the lacrimal duct, the surgeon can assess the integrity of the duct and either use this assessment for initial treatment by clearing any blockage present or for further surgical treatment. The surgeon uses a set of lacrimal probes which come in various graduated sizes — so as well as being used as an exploratory probe, they can be classed as a dilator. An example is the Bowman lacrimal probe (■ Figure 7.5).

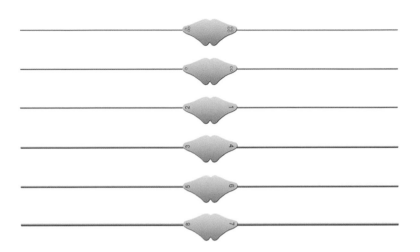

Figure 7.5. Bowman lacrimal probes.

Rigid endoscopes

For most diagnostic endoscopic procedures, a flexible endoscope can be used. These can access and examine the interior of a hollow organ, duct or cavity. As these will mainly be diagnostic, a biopsy specimen can also be taken or injections (for treatment) given through the flexible scope.

Rigid endoscopes, such as, for example, cystoscopes (■ Figure 7.6) (looking into the urinary bladder) or hysteroscopes (looking into the uterus) are used to perform specific procedures where a flexible scope would not be sufficient. Where, for example, a large resection is required, an endoscopic resectoscope would need to be used and this would be better performed through a rigid scope. An example is transurethral resection of the prostate (TURP). The resectoscope (■ Figure 7.7) is an instrument that consists of a sheath, normally fenestrated, that can accommodate a knife or electrosurgical cutting loop, as a working element, for surgery within a body cavity. The electrosurgical loop or knife may be either monopolar or bipolar — these may be single use or reusable and fit into the working element of the resectoscope (■ Figure 7.8).

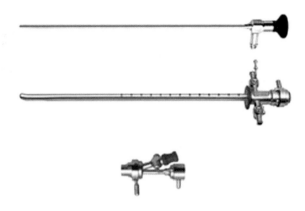

Figure 7.6. Rigid cystoscope.

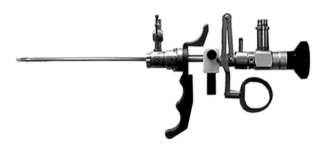

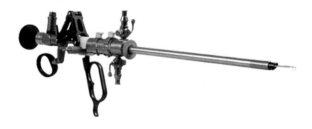

Figure 7.7. Resectoscopes.

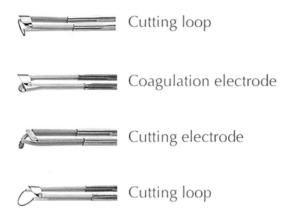

Figure 7.8. Bipolar electrosurgical resection instrument ends.

Other procedures that can be performed through an endoscope include the removal of renal stones (calculi) through ridged cystoscopy or ureteroscopy. Bladder stones can be removed in the same way but other, more specific devices are available to extract bladder stones. A retrieval system (Dormia-type basket) is passed into the ureter, opened around the stone, then closed to trap the stone, enabling extraction. ■ Figure 7.9 shows the process of inserting the catheter with the basket

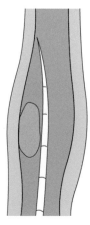
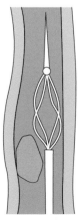
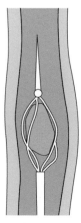

Figure 7.9. Removal of a renal stone from the ureter.

withdrawn inside the catheter, the basket device opening and capturing the stone, which is securely held prior to its removal. This is facilitated by direct vision through a rigid endoscope.

An example of a procedure that could be performed through a flexible endoscope is the removal of biliary stones in the proximal common bile duct. ■ Figure 7.10 shows the endoscope within the lumen of the duodenum and the stone retrieval basket being passed up the common bile duct (CBD) through a sphincterotomy to retrieve a biliary gallstone. The basket device is then withdrawn with the gallstone firmly grasped and held by the basket.

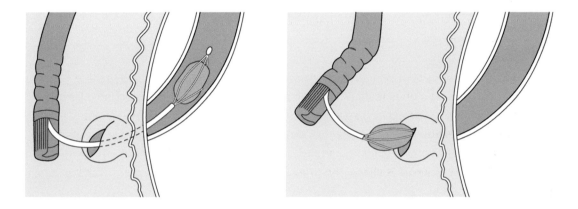

Figure 7.10. Biliary gallstone being removed from the CBD through a sphincterotomy.

Within this section it is worth mentioning instruments that are used to 'see' and 'observe' certain anatomical structures, or allow the surgeon to access areas he/she may need to operate through by proceeding through natural or surgically constructed orifices. These instruments are classed as speculums and perform a similar role to that of the retractor — they are discussed in more detail in Chapter 3 — "Retractors and speculums".

Briefly mentioned already is the dilator (lacrimal probe/dilator). These instruments are mentioned later in Chapter 8 — "Ancillary instrumentation".

Chapter 8

ANCILLARY INSTRUMENTATION

Instruments cannot always be categorised into specific design types or groups as they vary widely dependent upon the surgeon's preference of use, knowledge of instrumentation and hospital region. Instrument sets will differ and specific instruments within them will change. Some procedures require specific and unique instrumentation to facilitate with, or help, a specific procedure. In this chapter is an introduction to other instruments that are universally used but are not easily placed into function groups, for example, the Collingwood Stewart hernia ring (■ Figure 8.1) and the ligature pusher

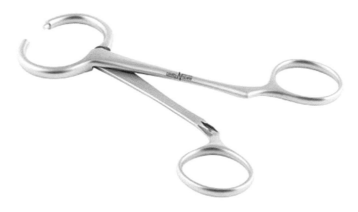

Figure 8.1. Collingwood Stewart hernia ring.

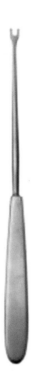

Figure 8.2. Negus ligature pusher.

(■ Figure 8.2). This chapter will also cover an overview of instruments in certain specialties.

Collingwood Stewart hernia ring

The Collingwood Stewart hernia ring (■ Figure 8.1) is an instrument designed to be placed around the inguinal cord during procedures performed within the inguinal canal. The 'ring' is placed around the inguinal cord so it can be manipulated and retracted to avoid damage to its vascular contents, as in the repair of an inguinal hernia where the surgeon defines the type of inguinal hernia present so a repair can be made.

A ligature pusher (■ Figure 8.2) is designed to aid knot tying and is a useful tool to aid the tying of ligatures or sutures in deep tissues, or anatomical areas where it would prove difficult for the surgeon to use his fingers to push the ligature sufficiently tight when knotting. The ENT surgeon would use this when tying ligatures around the tonsil vessels deep in the oropharynx during a tonsillectomy for example.

Aneurysm needle

An aneurysm needle (■ Figure 8.3), having a blunt or sharp point, is an instrument for suturing, puncturing or passing a suture or ligature around a structure such as an artery or vein to allow it to be tied off. The ligature is passed through the eye of the needle which is found at the point of the needle end of the instrument, pushed through and under the vessel and then captured on the other side by forceps allowing the surgeon to then tie it off.

Instruments for measurements

Surgeons may sometimes need to perform precisely measured interventions. These are done using a stainless steel ruler (■ Figure 8.4), or a pair of calipers (■ Figure 8.5). Measurements in surgery are important in many specialisms, including orthopaedic joint relacements, where specific measurements, sized jigs and trial instruments are used; ■ Figure 8.6 shows a femoral head-measuring device. In plastic and reconstructive surgery and maxillofacial surgery, reconstruction may need specific measurements in order to rebuild facial structures; so suitable and accurate measurements need to be made. In the case of ophthalmic procedures, a small pair of calipers can be used to measure distances in rectus muscle surgery (■ Figure 8.7), where resection and recession of these muscles need to be made in strabismus (squint) surgery.

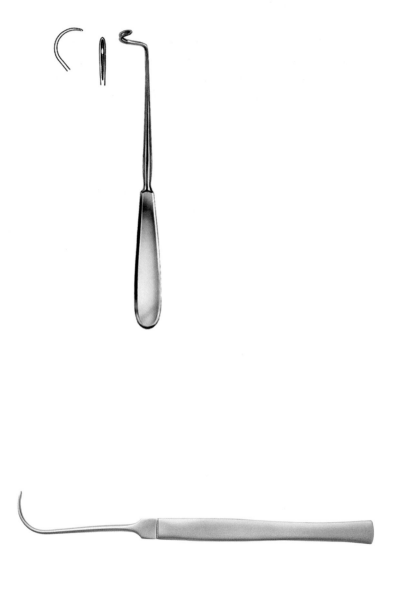

Figure 8.3. Syme aneurysm needle.

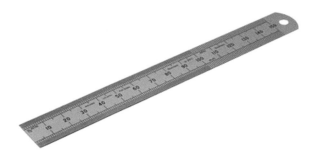

Figure 8.4. Stainless steel ruler.

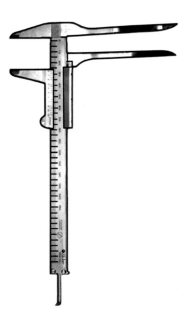

Figure 8.5. Orthopaedic calipers.

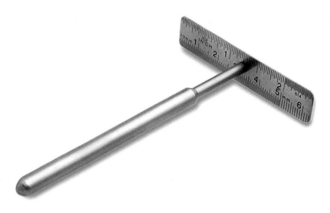

Figure 8.6. Femoral head-measuring device.

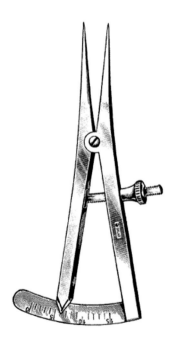

Figure 8.7. Castroviejo calipers.

The orthopaedic depth gauge (■ Figure 8.8) is designed to measure the appropriate screw length to fit a drilled hole in bone, to secure fractured bone fragments together or to allow a plate to be placed to repair a bone fracture or purpose-made bone cut or osteotomy.

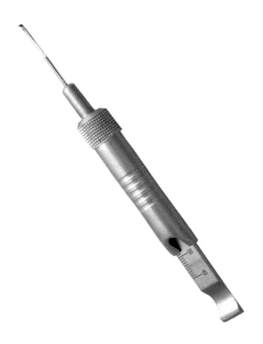

Figure 8.8. Orthopaedic depth gauge.

Uterine sound

A uterine sound is used to measure the internal depth of the uterus so perforation of the uterus is avoided when inserting other instruments, e.g. curettes and endoscopes. Two types to consider are the Sims (■ Figure 8.9) and Galabin (■ Figure 8.10) uterine malleable sound.

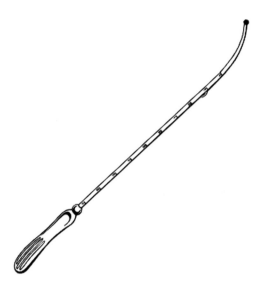

Figure 8.9. Sims uterine sound.

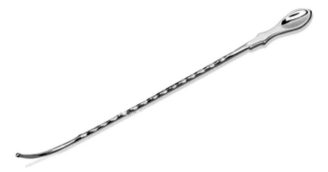

Figure 8.10. Galabin uterine sound.

Vascular instruments

The following show some of the basic vascular ancillary instruments that are used in vascular procedures to augment the general instruments that you would expect to find in a typical vascular set (other than the range of vascular clamps described earlier): the Cooley vascular measuring clamp (■ Figure 8.11), a vein stripper used in varicose vein surgery (■ Figure 8.12), a vascular shunt clamp (■ Figure 8.13) and vascular tunnelling devices for tunnelling grafts subcutaneously (■ Figure 8.14).

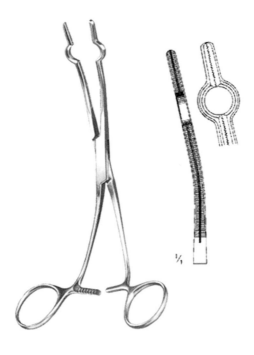

Figure 8.11. Vascular measuring clamp.

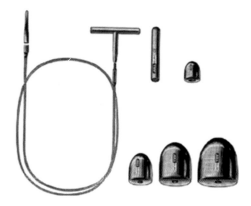

Figure 8.12. Vein stripper.

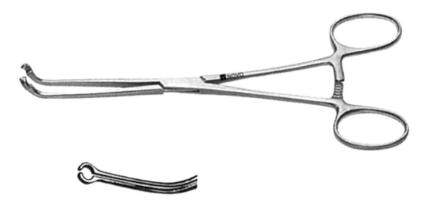

Figure 8.13. Vascular shunt clamp.

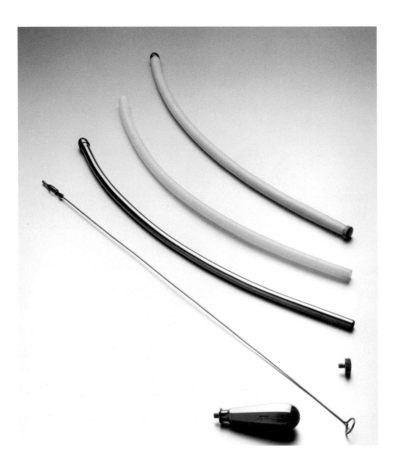

Figure 8.14. Vascular tunnelling device.

Phlebectomy hooks

Phlebectomy hooks (■ Figure 8.15) are instruments that are used to treat branch varicosities of the large and small saphenous veins. A series of small incisions or skin punctures are made in the skin over the varicosities and the hook is used to catch the vein and pull it through the incision where it is avulsed.

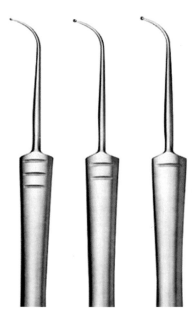

Figure 8.15. Phlebectomy hooks.

Tibbs flushing cannula

The Tibbs cannula (■ Figure 8.16) comes in various sizes with a 'peanut' or conical end providing a snug fit in a vessel which allows insertion into the blood vessel to flush it through with heparinised saline solution during vascular procedures.

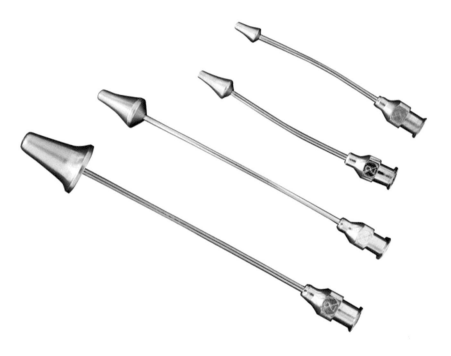

Figure 8.16. Tibbs cannula.

Biliary instruments

In biliary surgery, there may also be a requirement for Moynihan cholecystectomy forceps (■ Figure 8.17) or Lahey cholecystectomy duct forceps (■ Figure 8.18),

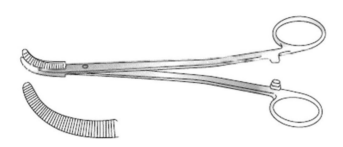

Figure 8.17. Moynihan cholecystectomy forceps.

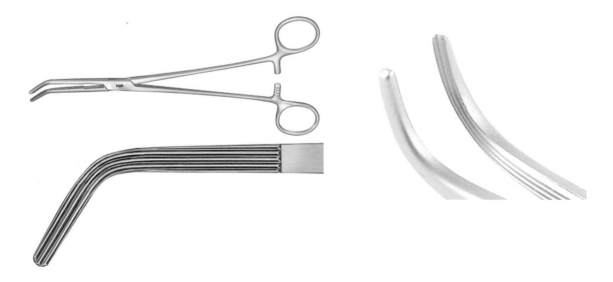

Figure 8.18. Lahey forceps showing the opened tips.

described earlier in Chapter 5 — "Clamps and clips". Lahey forceps may also be required by the vascular surgeon — so, clearly, some instruments have a number of roles and uses across a variety of specialties. They present in a number of sizes and lengths, some having fine tips and others slightly larger. These are versatile instruments that are used primarily for blunt dissection around vessels or ducts to identify them, and to pass ligatures or tapes around to facilitate their ligation or retraction. The angled and finer jaws make them an ideal instrument for this type of dissection. To manipulate or hold the gallbladder, the surgeon may use a pair of gallbladder lifting forceps — examples of which are the Mouat gallbladder lifting forceps or Judd Martel gallbladder forceps (■ Figure 8.19).

a   b

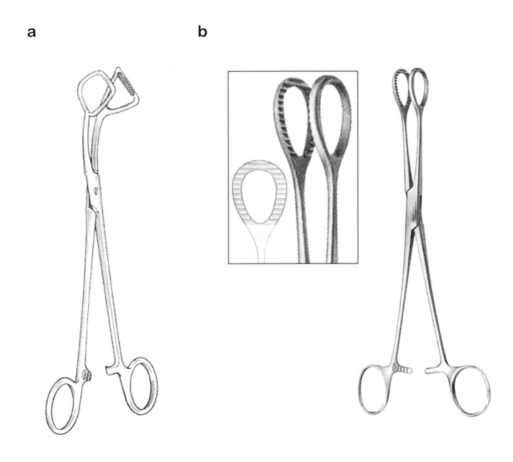

Figure 8.19. a) Mouat gallbladder lifting forceps. b) Judd Martel gallbladder forceps.

For exploring the common bile duct, a range of stone forceps or ductal exploration forceps are available to remove stones. This instrument is used to extract stones from the common bile duct. They can also be used to extract stones from the kidney, kidney pelvis and ureter. An example in common use is the Randall stone forceps which come with varying degrees of tip curvature (■ Figure 8.20).

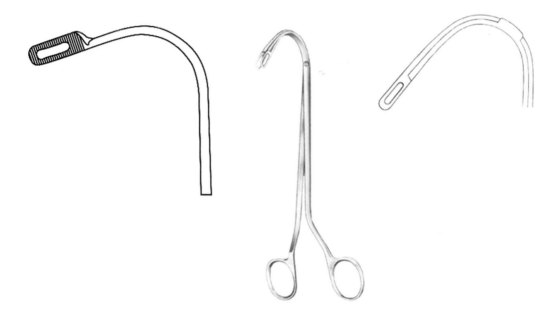

Figure 8.20. Randall stone forceps.

Micro instrumentation

Instruments that are used to perform microsurgery are usually small and delicate. They are precise devices that are normally used with operating microscopes or by surgeons using binocular loupes (■ Figure 8.21) to magnify the operative site. They allow the surgeon to manipulate and repair very small structures or tissue.

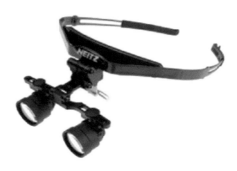

Figure 8.21. Binocular loupes.

Micro instruments, typically made of titanium or stainless steel (titanium being the preference as it is lighter in weight and stronger), maintain their edge and delicate precision in their active operating 'end'. The instrument finish is dull so light from the microscope is not reflected back into the eyes of the operating surgeon and his team. These instruments are designed to be manipulated with the thumb and forefinger which allows more subtle and delicate manoeuvres than would be otherwise achieved with instruments having ring finger handles; therefore, scissors and needle holders are operated with spring action handles (■ Figure 8.22) with a single ratchet that locks and unlocks the jaws of the needle holder through a single 'squeeze' of the instrument handle.

a

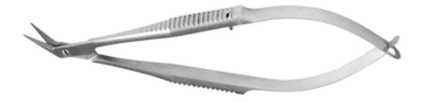

b

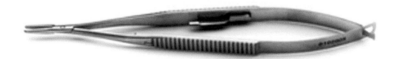

Figure 8.22. a) Spring scissors. b) Castroviejo needle holder.

Micro-thumb forceps used in ophthalmic surgery are small, delicate and have very fine points, as in a pair of Pierse-Hoskin forceps (■ Figure 8.23).

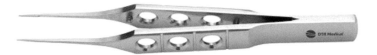

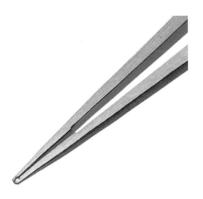

Figure 8.23. Pierse-Hoskin forceps showing the micro end.

In neurosurgery, the instruments are normally offset with an angle built into the handle. The arachnoid knife (■ Figure 8.24) is a commonly used knife for dissection with micro-dissectors and nerve hooks used for blunt dissection. Forceps (■ Figure 8.25) may have fine teeth or be plain or smooth, and may be curved or straight; they are also offset to aid vision when in use.

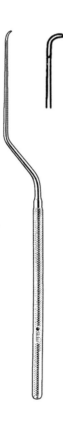

Figure 8.24. Arachnoid knife (showing the offset bend).

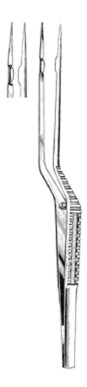

Figure 8.25. Micro forceps.

The fine ends and tips of these instruments need to be protected carefully because they are easily bent or thrown out of alignment if handled roughly.

Micro clips used with a clip applicator to occlude small vessels are also spring-loaded, as with the Yasargil clips (■ Figure 8.26). This technique of 'open surgical clipping' is performed for aneurysms in the vasculature of the brain to treat and prevent rupture of these aneurysms, which would cause a subarachnoid haemorrhage (■ Figure 8.27).

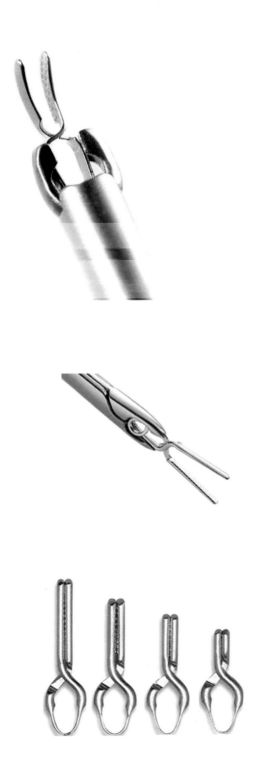

Figure 8.26. Yasargil clips.

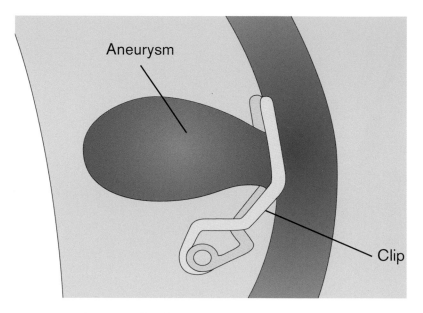

Figure 8.27. Application of a clip on an aneurysm.

Dilators

Dilators are instruments used to gradually dilate an orifice or duct to allow the introduction of a larger instrument, or to open a stricture in a duct or orifice. These dilators take the form and shape of the anatomical area in which they are to be used, such as urethral dilators, with different designs for males and females. The Clutton sound is an example of a male urethral dilator (■ Figure 8.28), and the Hegar dilator is an example of a female urethral dilator (■ Figure 8.29).

The Hegar female dilator gradually tapers from a wider proximal end to a thinner distal end and are found in a range of sizes. Some are single-ended whilst others are double-ended with the opposite end being one size up or down in its width.

Some dilators have been designed to dilate ducts, such as the Bakes dilator (■ Figure 8.30). The Bakes dilator has an oval tip of various sizes on a malleable shaft and can be used in choledocholithotomy to dilate the common bile duct, enabling stone removal. It can also be used to check the patency of the oesophagus in paediatric surgery and for probing the pancreatic duct and dilating the ampulla of Vater in cases of stricture.

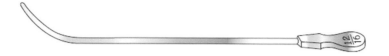

Figure 8.28. Clutton sound — male urethral dilator.

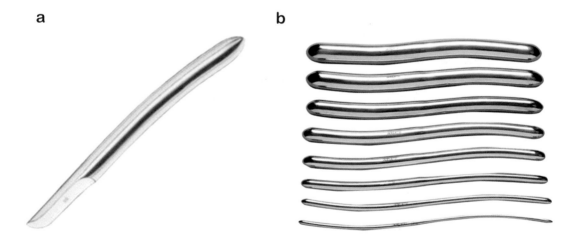

a

b

Figure 8.29. Hegar dilator — female dilator: a) single-ended; b) double-ended.

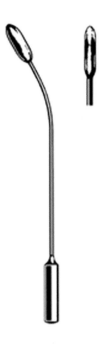

Figure 8.30. Bakes dilator.

The Nettleship dilator (■ Figure 8.31) is used to dilate the lacrimal punctum — usually in conjunction with the lacrimal probe to open the duct in the lacrimal sac, and to facilitate syringing to remove a blockage. ■ Figure 8.32 shows the Nettleship dilator in use to dilate the punctum.

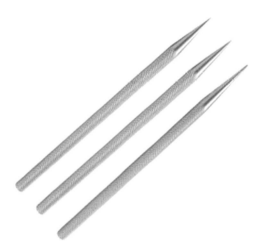

Figure 8.31. Nettleship dilator.

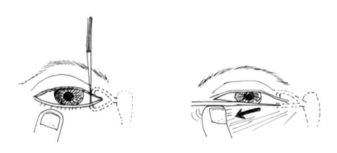

Figure 8.32. Dilatation of the lower eyelid punctum with a Nettleship dilator.

Cardiac dilators

An example of a specific cardiac dilator is the Tubbs transventricular dilator (■ Figure 8.33) for mitral valve stenosis. The instrument is used to open a closed or damaged mitral valve caused by age, disease or a defect that has been inherited. This still remains a popular instrument today even though it has been in use for a number of decades. When the Tubbs cardiac dilator instrument is passed into the mitral valve, the handle is closed, opening the dilator to 45mm in width.

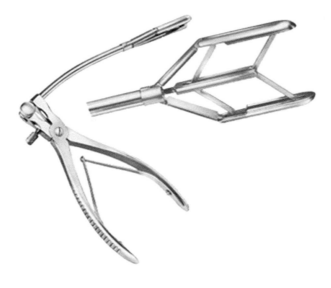

Figure 8.33. Tubbs cardiac dilator.

Sponge holder and towel clip

The sponge holder is another versatile instrument that is used primarily for holding swabs and sponges for 'prepping' the patient's skin prior to draping the operative site. It may also be used to grasp and manipulate structures or tissue without causing trauma or damage. Examples of its use in this role are in holding the gallbladder during an open cholecystectomy, and manipulating cervical tissue and removal of endometrial tissue during gynaecological procedures. A common use is for it to carry a fixed swab, known colloquially as a 'swab on a stick' to aid both blunt dissection and mopping up of blood. An example of a common sponge holder is the Rampley sponge holder (■ Figure 8.34) which is similar to the Foerster sponge holder (■ Figure 8.35).

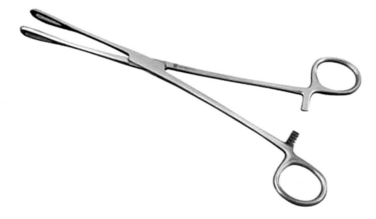

Figure 8.34. Rampley sponge holder.

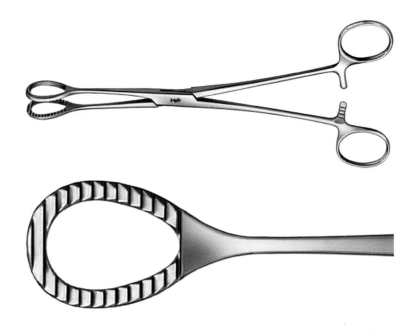

Figure 8.35. Foerster sponge holder.

Towel clips

The towel clip primarily was used to clip together the woven fabric drapes when isolating the operative site; however, most drapes in use today are made of disposable waterproof, impregnated paper fabric, which have an adhesive edge to hold them in position providing a secure seal around the operative site. Some surgeons when applying the towel clip to drapes used to clip them through the patient's skin, which in modern practice is thought to be inappropriate causing unnecessary damage. They can also be used to grasp tissue (and skin) to aid the surgeon's visualisation of wounds/structures and indeed they can be used to aid entry with a laparoscopic port. This use, to aid laparoscopic entry, is largely frowned upon in modern practice as it causes unnecessary skin damage. These towel clips or clamps have sharp, perforating tips as with the Backhaus towel clip or clamp (■ Figure 8.36). There are also towel clamps that have non-perforating tips such as the Lorna towel clamp (■ Figure 8.37) and clamps with a ball and socket tip (■ Figure 8.38). These will not perforate the towels and drape they are used to clamp.

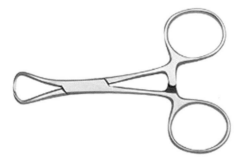

Figure 8.36. Backhaus towel clip.

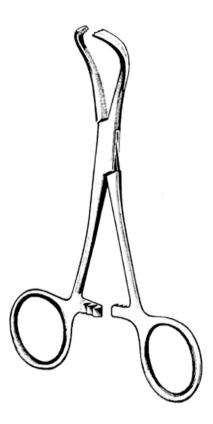

Figure 8.37. Lorna towel clamp.

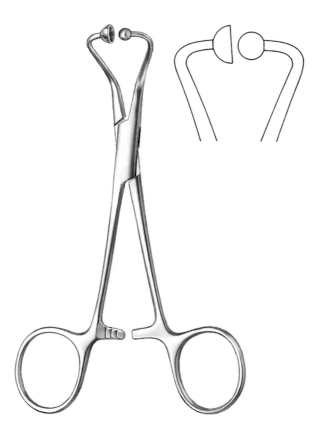

Figure 8.38. Towel clamp with a ball and socket tip.

Curettes

A curette or 'spoon' is an instrument designed to scrape or debride biological tissue from a number of various anatomical areas. They can be used to take tissue biopsies from the inside of body structures; for example, taking endometrial biopsies from the inside of the uterus. This is a hand tool that has a tip shaped as a spoon, hook or gouge to scrape and capture tissue for removal, with either blunt, but normally sharp, edges.

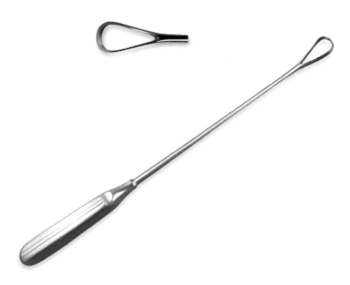

Figure 8.39. Curette loop.

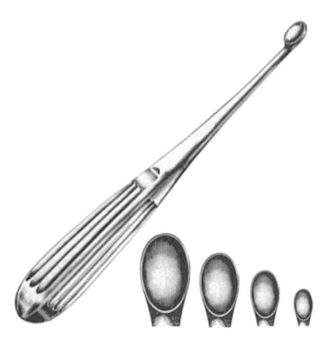

Figure 8.40. Curette spoon.

They can be used in a variety of ways and may be used to remove, for example, impacted ear wax, for the excision of adenoids (by scraping them out), for debriding abscesses and deroofing cysts to roughen the edges to promote healing and to take tissue for investigation. These are hand-held instruments that may be double-ended (with differing sized ends) or single-ended with a solid handle. ■ Figures 8.39, 8.40 and 8.41 show a variety of curettes.

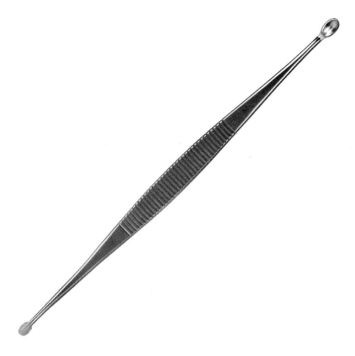

Figure 8.41. Volkmann spoon (curette).

Trocar (and cannula)

This is an instrument consisting of an obturator with a sharp cutting point and sharp edges at its distal end and a sheath or cannula (hollow tube) over the trocar that allows penetration of the skin or body cavity, leaving the cannula in place once the trocar has penetrated the structure and is removed. This may be for the drainage of fluid within that structure or for the insertion and placement of an endoscope. The trocar and cannula may be made of metal (■ Figure 8.42) or plastic with the trocar tip-bladed or non-bladed (■ Figure 8.43). The hollow cannula is normally left in place after tissue penetration. The function of this device in laparoscopic surgery is to allow passage of the operative telescope and instruments to facilitate surgery. The cannula has a seal so the pneumoperitoneum can be maintained. These 'ports' are discussed further in the laparoscopic instrument chapter — see Chapter 11.

Originally, surgeons used this device to drain fluid or gas from body cavities, as in abdominal ascites. Two examples of a trocar and cannula are shown below.

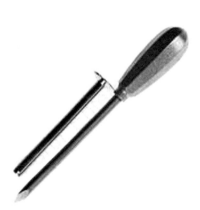

Figure 8.42. Trocar and cannula.

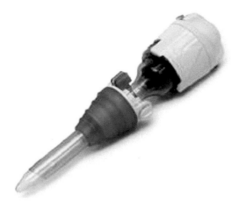

Figure 8.43. Laparoscopic first-entry cannula.

Dissectors

These instruments allow the surgeon to perform various blunt dissections of tissue within certain structures and are specifically designed for this purpose. An example in common use is the Watson-Cheyne dissector (■ Figure 8.44), which is a double-ended instrument that can be used both as a dissector and a probe; another double-ended instrument commonly used is the McDonald dissector (■ Figure 8.45), having a straight spade-type end and a curved end.

Some dissectors are designed to slip under specific structures to allow the surgeon to incise tissue over the instrument — the instrument therefore protects the anatomical structures and tissues underneath or behind the dissector. An example of this type is the Kocher thyroid dissector (■ Figure 8.46). This dissector has channels for the surgeon to cut down onto giving some direction and protection to the cut.

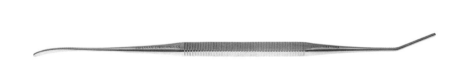

Figure 8.44. Watson-Cheyne dissector.

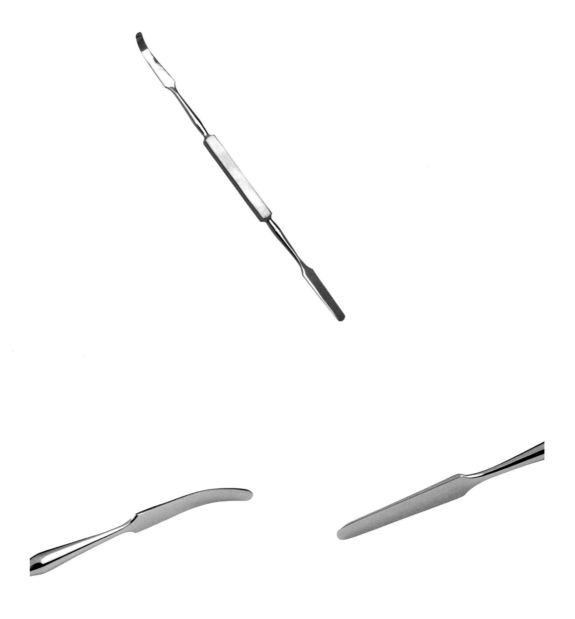

Figure 8.45. McDonald dissector showing the two different ends.

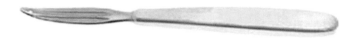

Figure 8.46. Kocher thyroid dissector.

Chapter 9

INTESTINAL INSTRUMENTS

Intestinal instruments are added to general and major laparotomy sets of instruments to facilitate specific surgery on small and large intestine and include clamps needed to occlude bowel to prevent leakage of bowel content. They include extra-long forceps, stapling devices and intraluminal devices such as the Poole-type suction cannula/tips (described earlier in Chapter 6 — "Suction devices") and intestinal decompression instruments, such as the Savage decompressor (■ Figure 9.1), based on a trocar and cannula design — the sharp trocar penetrates and introduces the cannula into the bowel that requires decompressing, and suction is applied to the cannula to evacuate the build-up of air.

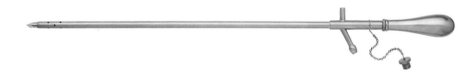

Figure 9.1. Savage decompressor.

Bowel clamps

A variety of bowel clamps are needed to facilitate both bowel occlusion and bowel crushing, used for resection and refashioning of bowel. Occlusion clamps such as the Doyen bowel clamp (■ Figure 9.2) are non-crushing and are designed to be used on bowel not to be damaged, whereas the crushing type of clamp will crush only bowel tissue that is due to be resected. These instruments hold bowel more securely and will, by crushing the bowel held, damage the bowel tissue. Examples of crushing clamps are the Payr and Parker-Kerr clamps (■ Figure 9.3). The Parker-Kerr clamp

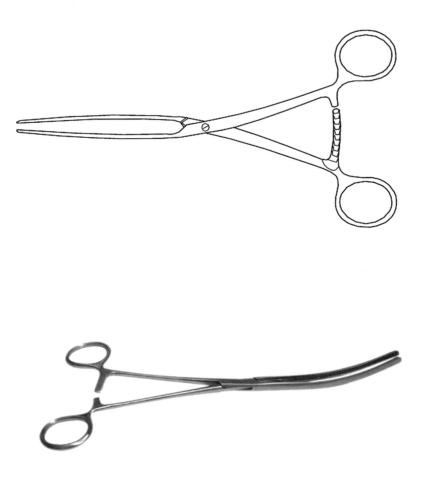

Figure 9.2. Non-crushing Doyen occlusion bowel clamp.

a

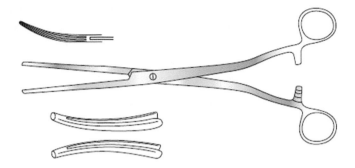

b

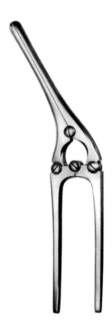

Figure 9.3. a) Parker-Kerr clamp with jaw shields. b) Payr clamp.

has a slotted shield that fits over the jaws of the clamp; once applied, it secures the clamp jaws and protects from bowel seepage getting into the abdomen.

The Lane twin anastomosis clamp (■ Figure 9.4) was originally designed for stomach resection and has two sets of clamps that can be joined together, allowing resected stomach to be approximated, aiding the reanastomosis. It can be used both on small and large bowel in the same way. The Lane twin anastomosis clamp is a non-crushing clamp.

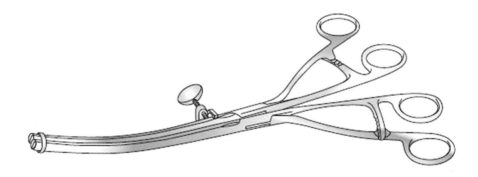

Figure 9.4. Lane twin anastomosis clamp.

Stapling devices

Surgical stapling devices (■ Figure 9.5) have revolutionised gastrointestinal surgery both for open and laparoscopic procedures. They have made the formation of anastomoses much quicker, simpler and more secure for every part of the gastrointestinal tract.

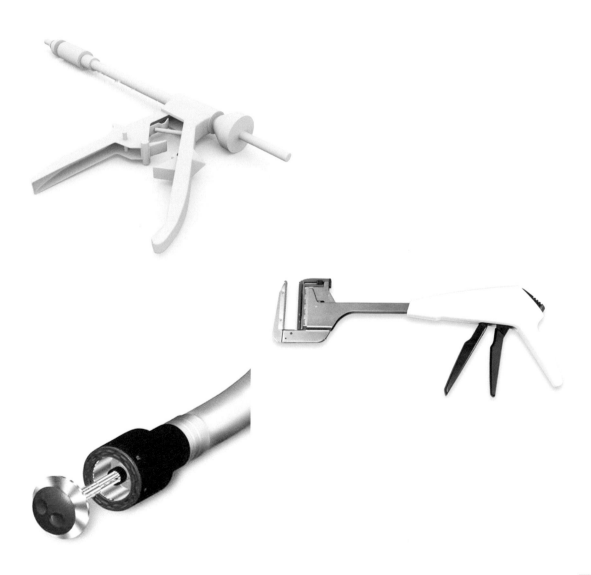

Figure 9.5. Stapling devices.

The stapling device was initiated as a mechanical suturing device that allows for a superior result in end-to-end anastomoses, in comparison to that of hand suturing. It causes less trauma than manual suturing and performs an end-to-end intestinal anastomosis (■ Figure 9.6) that is superior and more anatomically sound. The forerunners were cylindrical devices that resembled a proctoscope and could be inserted peranally, so making resection of lower colonic and rectal tumours more anatomically sound, obviating the need for a permanent colostomy, as the descending/transverse colon could be rejoined or anastomosed to the remaining rectal or anal stump. This proved ideal as the traditional abdominoperineal resection was the operation of choice and usually resulted in closure of the anus with a resultant permanent colostomy. Hand suturing of colon to the rectum or anal stump is difficult or almost impossible.

The instrument is cylindrical in shape with a cone that can be opened away from and subsequently closed onto the main barrel of the instrument. The proximal and distal ends of the remaining bowel, after the main resection has taken place, are secured around the 'nose cone' and barrel of the device onto the shaft and then drawn together to approximate them. The device is then 'fired' by squeezing the handle which inserts a cylindrical row of staples into both ends of the bowel and simultaneously cuts two discs of bowel from the lumen inside the stapled ends.

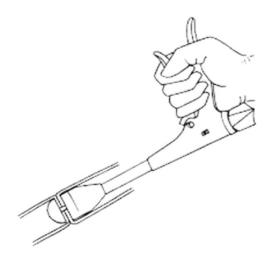

Figure 9.6. The principle of the stapling gun in an end-to-end anastomosis.

These resemble 'doughnuts' in shape and allow the surgeon to see that two complete rings of tissue have been taken, proving that a sound anastomosis has been formed.

The circular stapler has also been used successfully to treat haemorrhoids (■ Figure 9.7). It provides a quick and accurate solution with a faster recovery for patients who present with haemorrhoids, or prolapse, having a unique advantage over that of conventional surgical excision as it is used above the dentate line inside the anal canal. The stapler is applied in the anal canal for transection and resection of internal tissue affecting fewer nerve endings, therefore providing a procedure which is less painful.

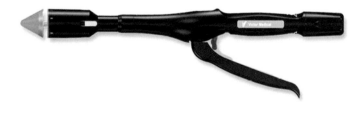

Figure 9.7. Disposable haemorrhoidal stapler.

Anterior resection of the rectum

A stapling gun inserted via the rectum and used to anastomose rectum to large bowel after resection is shown in ■ Figure 9.8. The circular stapler has made this procedure much easier and produces a more secure suture line with a circular row of double staples. This produces an end-to-end anastomosis (EEA) between the bowel and rectum.

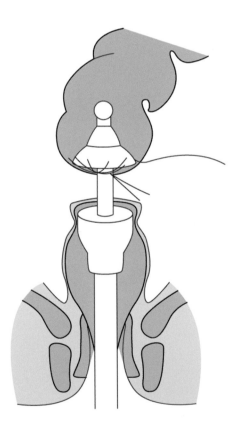

Figure 9.8. Stapling gun inserted through the anus to anastomose distal colon showing a purse-string suture in place.

The development of stapling devices has now progressed into minimally invasive surgery and/or laparoscopic procedures (■ Figure 9.9). Interest has been generated as laparoscopic surgery has developed and the development of laparoscopic linear cutters and staplers has allowed the surgeon to perform upper and lower gastrointestinal procedures, colectomies, gastric surgery and, more recently, surgery for bariatric cases through this route.

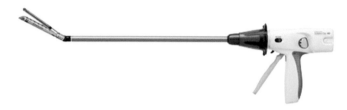

Figure 9.9. Laparoscopic stapling device.

Chapter 10

GYNAECOLOGICAL INSTRUMENTS

A variety of specialised instruments are available to the gynaecologist that will cover open abdominal, vaginal and laparoscopic procedures. The instruments used will vary between different regional theatres and the surgeon's preferences for his/her own practice. The following provides information on the more commonly used instruments and their uses; speculums have been covered in Chapter 3 — "Retractors and speculums", and dilators have been covered in Chapter 8 — "Ancillary instrumentation".

Uterine sound

A uterine sound is a long instrument with some malleability in its shaft, having a blunt tip to avoid perforation to the uterine wall. It has measurements on the shaft to gauge the depth of the uterine cavity and length of the cervix. It can also be used to feel for any specific pathology within the uterine cavity such as fibroids or anatomical abnormalities like a uterine septum or a bicornuate uterus. They are commonly found on dilatation and curettage sets (D&C). An example of a uterine sound is the Galabin (■ Figure 10.1) or Sims (■ Figure 10.2) uterine sound.

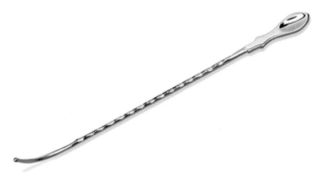

Figure 10.1. Galabin uterine sound.

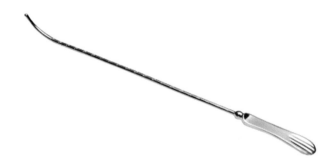

Figure 10.2. Sims uterine sound.

Tenaculum forceps

These instruments are used for grasping the cervix, usually at the anterior/superior lip of the cervix. The vulsellum forceps usually has three to four teeth and are very sharp. The tenaculum is a straight instrument and has only a single sharp point at the tip (■ Figure 10.3). Both instruments are employed to hold and steady the cervix

a   b

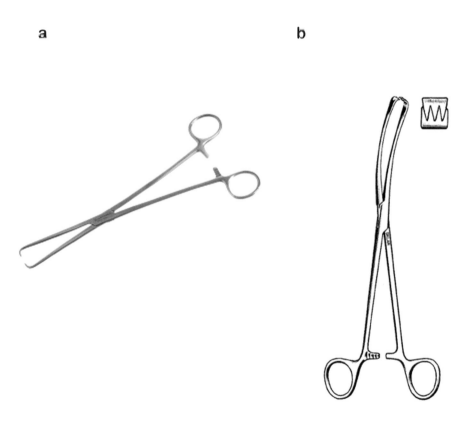

Figure 10.3. a) Tenaculum forceps. b) Vulsellum forceps.

when performing procedures such as the insertion of a uterine sound, a cervical biopsy, a vaginal hysterectomy, insertion of a Spackman cannula (■ Figure 10.4) (for laparoscopic gynaecological procedures) or any hysteroscopic procedure. The vulsellum forceps being extremely sharp are not used if there is a potential danger of tearing the cervix.

Spackman cannula

The Spackman cannula (■ Figure 10.4) is inserted into the opening of the cervix and is secured in place by either tenaculum or vulsellum forceps, the handle rings of

a

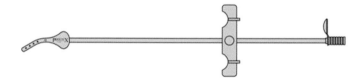

b

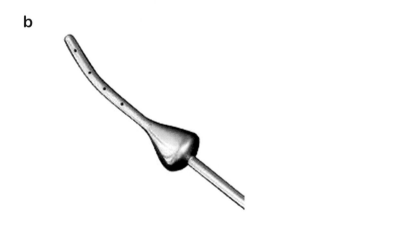

Figure 10.4. a) Spackman cannula. b) Cannula tip.

the forceps being attached to the manoeuvrable, hooked plate on the shaft. The Spackman cannula is used for injecting methylene blue dye for laparoscopic hysterosalpingography to check the patency of the Fallopian tubes in suspected tubal blockage. It is also placed *in situ* for laparoscopic procedures to enable manipulation of the uterus as the surgeon looks into the abdominal pelvis. The uterus can be retroverted, anteverted, or moved laterally, so the surgeon can see all aspects of the anatomy.

Episiotomy scissors

Episiotomy scissors are used to perform an episiotomy prior to a vacuum or forceps delivery. The scissors are shaped so the bottom blade (■ Figure 10.5) is inserted in the vagina whilst the baby's head is protected by the practitioner's fingers, as the procedure is performed when the baby's head crowns. Normally the episiotomy is done as a mediolateral cut which can be extended to the anus if a median approach is adopted.

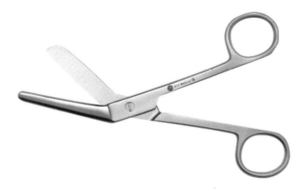

Figure 10.5. Episiotomy scissors.

Polyp forceps

This instrument may be straight or curved and is used to retrieve intrauterine polyps. The cervix is normally dilated sufficiently to allow passage and opening of the instrument to grasp any polyps within the uterus (■ Figure 10.6). It is similar in design to the sponge holder but with smaller jaws. The sponge holder can sometimes be the instrument of choice if there are large polyps to retrieve. Its insertion is dependent upon how wide the cervix can be dilated. An example of polyp forceps is the Bonney forceps (■ Figure 10.7).

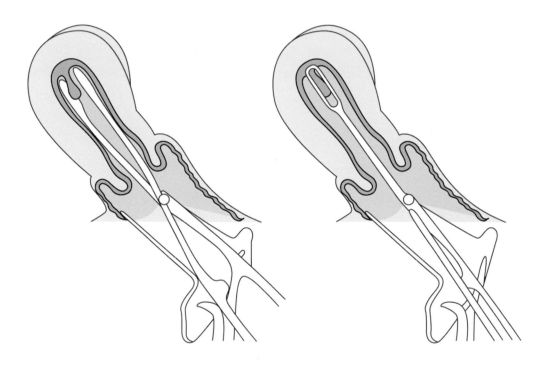

Figure 10.6. Uterine forceps in use, shown grasping an intrauterine polyp.

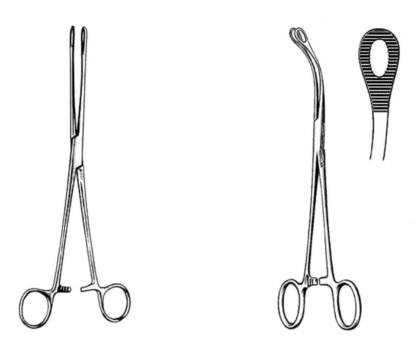

Figure 10.7. Polyp forceps (Bonney).

Vaginal wall retractors

Both the Landon (■ Figure 10.8) and Sims (■ Figure 10.9) retractors can be used in conjunction with the Sims or Auvard speculum making it easier to visualise the cervix and vagina. They are especially useful for anterior and posterior vaginal repairs for a cystocoele, enterocoele and rectocoele.

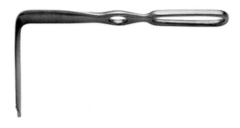

Figure 10.8. Landon anterior vaginal wall retractor.

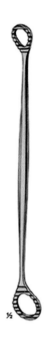

Figure 10.9. Sims anterior vaginal wall retractor.

Gynaecological clamps

Kocher forceps (■ Figure 10.10) (or clamp) are a commonly used instrument in gynaecological surgery due to their robust holding features. They are used to clamp and hold the major vascular pedicles in hysterectomy and both straight and curved on flat instruments are used in tandem. Any pedicle or vascular tissue can be held

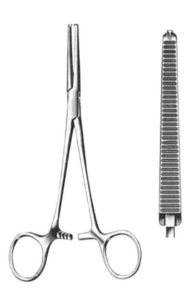

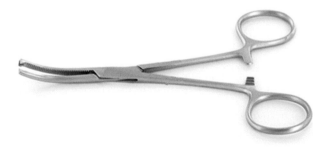

Figure 10.10. Kocher (Ochsner) forceps.

securely in the jaws which have teeth at the tips — these add security when tissue is grasped. Other specific clamps, such as the Gwilliam hysterectomy clamp (■ Figure 10.11), Heaney-Ballentine hysterectomy clamp (■ Figure 10.12) and Maingot hysterectomy clamp (■ Figure 10.13) are designed for grasping the uterine tissue and pedicles to facilitate excision and ligation. This is very thick, muscular tissue containing major vessels which requires a firm, secure hold. If this hold slips there could be a massive haemorrhage which may be difficult to control — hence a very robust, toothed clamp is required.

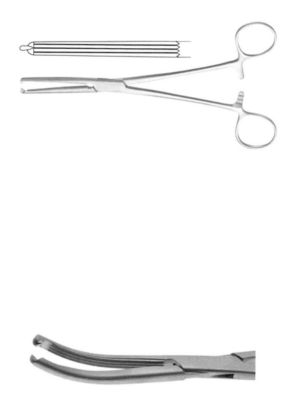

Figure 10.11. Gwilliam hysterectomy clamp.

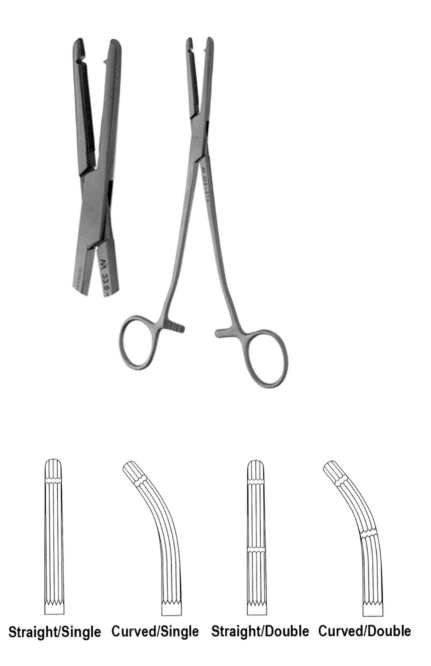

Straight/Single   Curved/Single   Straight/Double   Curved/Double

Figure 10.12. Heaney-Ballentine hysterectomy clamp.

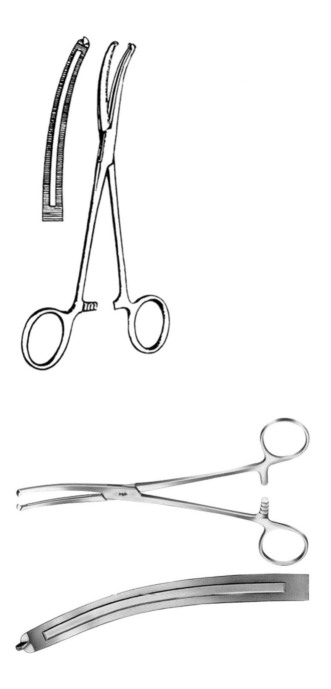

Figure 10.13. Maingot hysterectomy clamp.

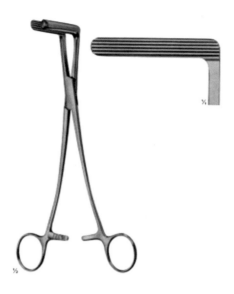

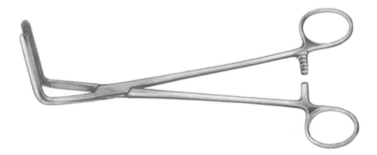

Figure 10.14. Wertheim vaginal and pedicle clamp.

These abdominal hysterectomy clamps, like the Kocher forceps, are designed to grasp and hold vascular pedicles firmly, as inadvertent 'slippage' of the pedicle from the instrument could result in major and catastrophic haemorrhage. These instruments are robust and are presented with various designs of jaw serrations/inserts and teeth, to firmly hold tissue in between them. For vaginal pedicles, the Wertheim pedicle clamp (■ Figure 10.14) is the instrument of choice.

Elevating forceps

Uterine elevating forceps, such as the Somer forceps (■ Figure 10.15), are commonly use to extract tumours, tissue or polyps from the uterus by elevating the vaginal wall. The jaws are serrated to allow a firm hold when grasping the tissue to be removed and they are curved to allow full visualisation during the procedure. The uterine elevator is also useful in manoeuvring the uterine wall, making the removal of tissue easier.

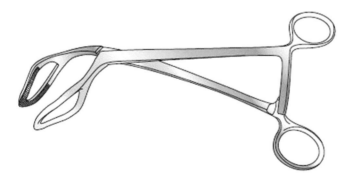

Figure 10.15. Somer uterine elevating forceps.

Myomectomy screw

To facilitate the removal of a fibroid tumour from within the uterine wall, it may be necessary to securely hold the fibroid and manipulate it, whilst excising it from the myometrium, the muscle layer of the uterus. The myomectomy screw is 'screwed' into the fibroid which allows a firm hold on the tissue as the surgeon dissects it out. It can be used for both open, abdominal procedures and also for laparoscopic excision, using a smaller 5mm instrument (■ Figure 10.16) enabling passage down a 5mm port.

a   **b**

c

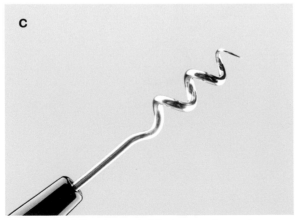

Figure 10.16. a) and b) Large (open) myomectomy screw. c) Laparoscopic myomectomy screw.

Cervical biopsy

The surgeon will sometimes need to remove a small amount of tissue from the cervix if any abnormality is suspected (usually found on routine examination or Pap smear).

This tissue is removed for histological examination, and the extent of abnormal tissue to be examined and removed will dictate the instruments used for this procedure. Punch biopsy forceps normally suffice for this procedure (■ Figure 10.17), but more extensive excision may need a cone biopsy, whereby a circular,

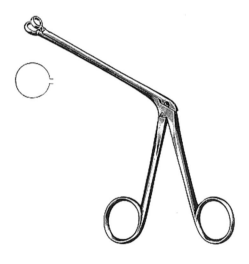

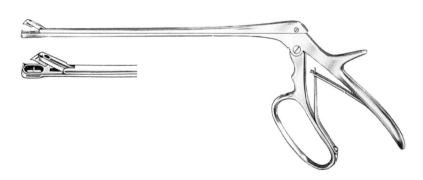

Figure 10.17. Cervical biopsy forceps.

cone-shaped piece of tissue is taken to include the opening of the cervix. This is normally facilitated by scalpel or laser excision (■ Figure 10.18).

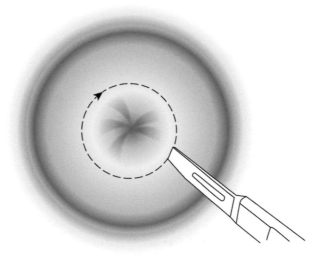

Figure 10.18. Scalpel excision for cone biopsy showing the incision route.

Chapter 11

LAPAROSCOPIC INSTRUMENTS

One of the most recent developments to have revolutionised surgery is the development of minimally invasive, keyhole, laparoscopic surgery. Even though the framework of laparoscopic surgery has been developed from over a century ago, modern techniques have been a rapidly growing science since the 1960s and 1970s, when it became a vital part of gynaecologists' practice. Since that time it has become fully integrated into the armamentarium of the general surgeon. This followed the development of the video chip and camera which placed the images onto the television screen, allowing for magnification and wider observation of the operative site.

Modern developments have allowed high definition and 3-D imaging, hand-assisted laparoscopic surgery (HALS)(■ Figure 11.1), and the use of 'single-port' laparoscopic surgery (SPLS) (■ Figure 11.2).

Single-port laparoscopic surgery, being one of the latest advances, allows the surgeon to use flexible endoscopes and articulating instruments. The surgeon can perform complex procedures through one single, or multiple, small incisions in the abdomen, into which he/she can place the telescope and the operating instruments. The main incision is normally made at the umbilicus; as with the normal multi-port technique, the scar can be hidden within this area. The number of operations that can

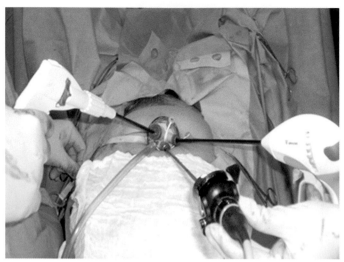

Figure 11.1. Single entry port in use showing instrument and camera placements.

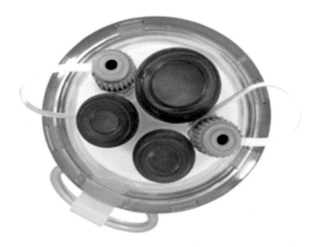

Figure 11.2. Single port showing a three-port entry facility and two gas entry ports, for single-port laparoscopic surgery (SPLS).

be performed laparoscopically are now multiple and have replaced the need for a large abdominal incision, such as:

- Nephrectomy.
- Prostatectomy.
- Hemicolectomy.
- Cholecystectomy.
- Splenectomy.
- Intussusception reduction.
- Gastrostomy tube placement and appendectomy.

In gynaecology, SPLS has been used to perform:

- Oophorectomy.
- Salpingectomy.
- Bilateral tubal ligation.
- Ovarian cystectomy.
- Surgical treatment of ectopic pregnancy.
- Both total and partial hysterectomy.

Laparoscopes

The modern 'telescope' has been adapted to carry light through fibreoptics and to magnify through a series of lenses, allowing the surgeon to view structures at different angles to facilitate the procedure within the abdomen. They normally provide a 0°, 12°, 30° and 70° angle of vision (■ Figure 11.3). The image is digitised through the camera processor where it can undergo some additional processing, such as filtering, 'noise' reduction, image enhancement and colour adjustment. This image is then sent to the monitor where it can be viewed not only by the surgeon but by the rest of the surgical team. Some telescopes have a flexible end that can be manipulated by the surgeon to obtain a view from a number of angles rather than by just 'set' angles (■ Figure 11.4).

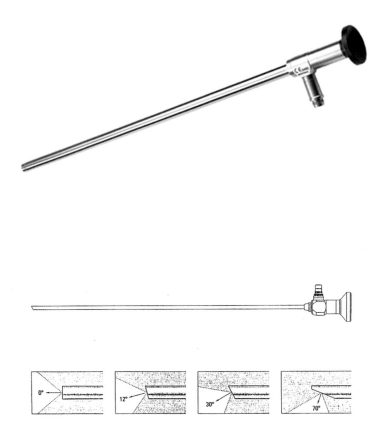

Figure 11.3. Telescope: 10mm laparoscope showing the various angles for viewing.

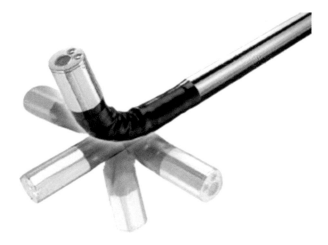

Figure 11.4. Flexible-ended telescope.

Light cables

There are two main types of light cables available to connect the telescope to the light source on the stack system: fluid-filled cables and fibreoptic cables. Fluid-filled cables tend to conduct more heat than fibreoptic cables and are usually stiffer in nature, so they are a little more difficult to manipulate and manoeuvre. Some have an inability to be autoclaved, so sterilisation becomes an issue.

Fibreoptic cables (■ Figure 11.5) are more user-friendly and more flexible, but are more fragile, so if roughly handled are prone to damage. If the fibres break and become greater than 25% damaged, then the cable should be replaced as the diminished light transmission will adversely affect the vision of the operative site.

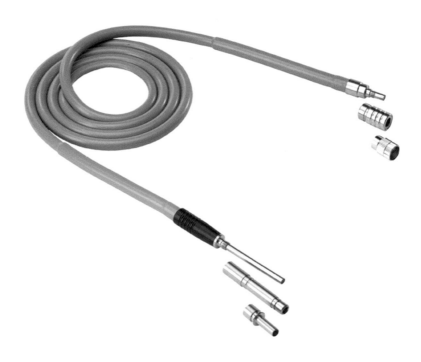

Figure 11.5. Typical light lead with multiple connectors.

Trocars and ports

There are many types and designs of laparoscopic trocars available — some reusable (■ Figure 11.6) and most, in modern practice, are disposable, single use (■ Figure 11.7). Some have an integral shielded blade to aid insertion, whilst some have

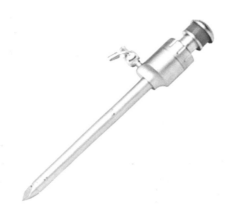

Figure 11.6. Reusable metal port.

a   **b**

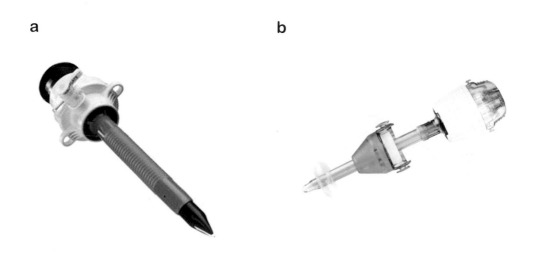

Figure 11.7. Laparoscopic ports: a) 10mm first entry; b) 5mm with a retaining balloon.

a sharp plastic point or a blunt point. The trocars are referred to as 'initial' or first-entry ports and secondary-entry ports. The first-entry ports, which are normally placed to take the telescope, are 10mm or 12mm diameter ports. The 5mm port is inserted as a secondary entry; these will take the operating instruments. All the ports have a one-way silicone or rubber seal which helps to maintain the pneumoperitoneum when the scope or instrument is removed. Some first-entry ports allow the telescope to be placed inside as the port trocar as it is being introduced, to allow the surgeon to visualise its entry into the abdomen — thus reducing the danger of damaging abdominal contents. The port hub has a small entry port with a control tap that allows the insufflation tubing to be attached.

Hand-assisted laparoscopic surgery (HALS)

The surgeon uses his/her non-dominant hand to guide and manipulate the laparoscopic instruments in this variation of laparoscopic surgery. By using his/her hand, it allows a greater flexibility and sensory feel to the procedure which ultimately makes the operation safer, giving a greater depth of feel and touch to guide his/her dissection. It also allows retraction of tissue and structures that would otherwise not be feasible when using instrument retractors. It has a greater advantage in some procedures, where larger organs are excised, such as the spleen, by allowing the organ or structure to be removed from the abdomen whole rather than piecemeal. The hand access port, such as the GelPort® (■ Figure 11.8),

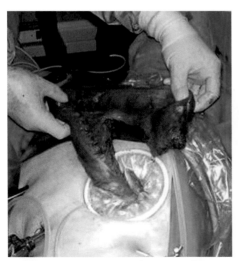 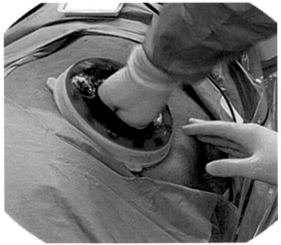

Figure 11.8. HALS technique showing port position and colon removal through the port.

allows the pneumoperitoneum to remain intact whilst the hand is inside the abdomen.

The HALS technique can be used to perform a number of different procedures through smaller incisions, such as:

- Colectomy (hemicolectomy or anterior resection).
- Hepatectomy.
- Splenectomy.
- Nephrectomy.
- Gastrectomy.

Insufflation of the abdomen

Entry into the abdomen with a port is a blind technique and does present problems with a number of possible complications, for example, the surgeon may perforate the bowel, liver or a major blood vessel. To help overcome this, there are two main recognised entry methods. The classic technique, still used today by many gynaecologists, is by using a Veress needle to insufflate the abdomen before entering with a port. The other is the classic open technique, or Hasson technique, where the surgeon makes an incisional opening, identifying structures through their layers down to the peritoneum before inserting the port, before inflating the abdomen. In both techniques, the abdomen is then inflated with carbon dioxide gas.

The Veress needle has an external diameter of 2mm with an external, sharp hypodermic-like point. Internally there is a spring-loaded inner cannula that has a blunt point which when the resistance of the abdominal wall is overcome on entering the abdominal cavity, springs forward so just the inner blunt atraumatic cannula is exposed. This blunt tip is designed to prevent entry into abdominal contents.

The Veress needles in use now are mainly single use (■ Figure 11.9); however, multiple use ones are still available (■ Figure 11.10). The normal entry point for the Veress needle is through the umbilicus.

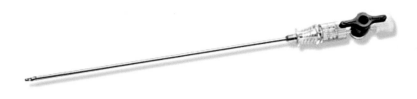

Figure 11.9. Veress needle — disposable.

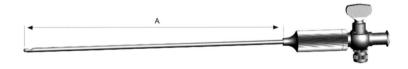

Figure 11.10. Veress needle — the reusable length (A) is normally 12-15cm.

Laparoscopic instruments

The instruments used are often miniature variations of the normal general surgical instruments used in open surgery. The tips of the instruments are smaller versions of their larger counterparts, and as such they are able to do the following:

- Aspirate.
- Dissect.
- Grasp.
- Retract.
- Cut, clip and staple.
- Suture.
- Cauterise using monopolar and bipolar electrosurgery.

The instrument design requirements are based upon the procedure being performed through a small incision, and with a lack of direct open vision. They are designed to provide the ergonomic conditions for the surgeon to manipulate them single-handed, operating all the functions of the instrument with one hand. The instruments must be light, but robust and comfortable in the surgeon's hand to allow repetitive movement over prolonged periods of time; some of which requires a delicate touch, especially in long dissection.

The instruments have rounded edges and have darkened surfaces to reduce reflected light. Most instruments need to be covered in an insulating coating so electrocautery may be used at the tip of the instrument without causing thermal damage to surrounding organs or tissue.

Each 'hand' instrument is usually around 30-33cm long and their main parts are:

- Handles — with and without a ratchet device, some with an electrode connector (■ Figure 11.11).
- Rotator device, usually attached to the handle, to allow a full 360° rotation of the working instrument tip.
- The shaft which should be insulated.
- Inner operative/working part.

The instruments should be easy to assemble and disassemble with the parts being interchangeable between similar instruments. They should have a simple design with minimal hinges/bolts and should be easy to clean and sterilise.

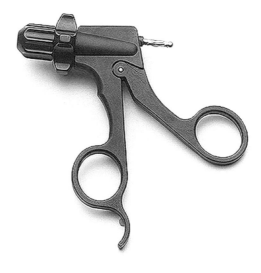

Figure 11.11. Laparoscopic handle (non-ratchet).

A number of differing instrument tips are available to aid the surgeon to perform specific tasks and to grasp various types of tissue — most are similar in design to the larger general instruments used in open surgery but are obviously smaller and slimmer to facilitate the keyhole approach. Examples of such instruments are shown below. There are fenestrated atraumatic graspers, the Johan fenestrated graspers (■ Figure 11.12). Others include a myoma screw, scissors and curved graspers (■ Figure 11.13). Another frequently used tip is the Maryland curved dissector (■ Figure 11.14), which is commonly used with diathermy attached to secure haemostasis. Some have a heavy toothed design to hold and grasp tissue securely and others have an atraumatic end such as the Babcock graspers for holding delicate tissue such as bowel. Examples can be seen in ■ Figure 11.15. One of the most used and useful instruments to help with dissection is the 'L' or 'J' diathermy hook (■ Figure 11.16).

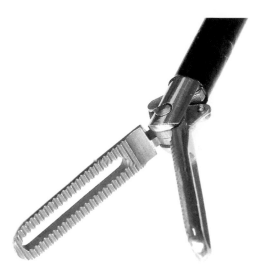

Figure 11.12. Atraumatic fenestrated tip (Johan).

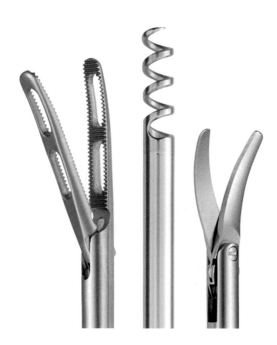

Figure 11.13. Instrument tips — grasper, myoma screw and scissors.

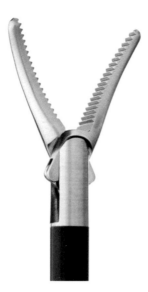

Figure 11.14. Maryland dissector tip.

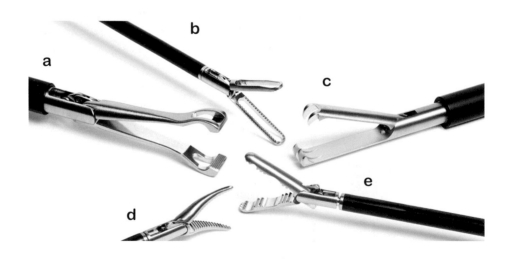

Figure 11.15. Multiple instrument tips showing various graspers: a) Babcock grasper. b) Johan (fenestrated) grasper. c) Heavy toothed grasper. d) Maryland grasper. e) Serrated alligator toothed grasper.

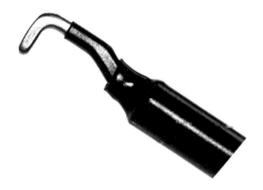

Figure 11.16. Laparoscopic diathermy 'L' hook showing insulation up to the working tip.

Laparoscopic needle holders with a ring and axial handle

Laparoscopic suturing is probably the most difficult procedure of any laparoscopic operation. It requires great dexterity and must be mastered by every laparoscopic surgeon; one of the most difficult acts is that of knot tying which requires the knot to be secure and safe with appropriate 'tightness' that can generally only be achieved with instrument tying — unless using a HALS approach when it can be aided by the surgeon's hand. A laparoscopic ligature pusher can also be used through a separate port. These instruments vary in design; some have ring handles and others have palm grip axial handles. The tips of laparoscopic needle holders (■ Figure 11.17), resemble normal needle holders with some having a tungsten carbide insert, as normal hand-held needle holders would have.

A common technique used to provide haemostasis during laparoscopic procedures and ligation where suturing would normally be used in open surgery, is the use of laparoscopic clips. A number of clipping devices are available to the surgeon. Clips are made primarily of titanium and are placed onto vessels and structures that need to be divided, sealed and dissected (■ Figure 11.18).

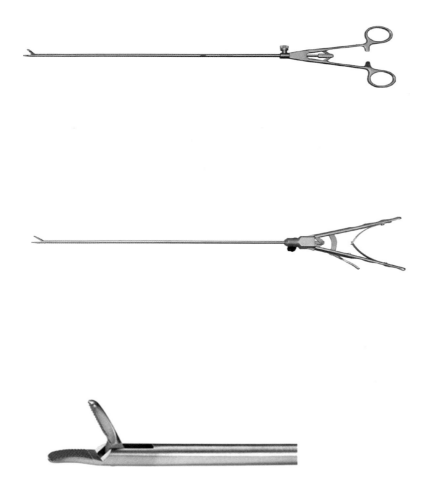

Figure 11.17. Laparoscopic needle holders with tips showing the tungsten insert.

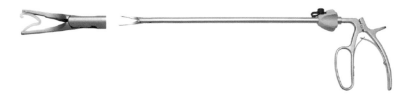

Figure 11.18. Laparoscopic clipper using locking clips.

A common use is in laparoscopic cholecystectomy where the cystic duct and cystic artery are divided prior to removal of the gallbladder (■ Figure 11.19).

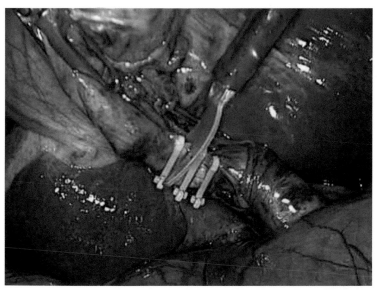

Figure 11.19. Division of the cystic duct after clipping with locking clips.

Laparoscopic retractors

One of the main problems encountered by the laparoscopic surgeon is good visual access to the operative site when other structures, such as bowel or the stomach, or any other overlying organ or tissue, obliterate the view. A number of different laparoscopic retractors (■ Figure 11.20) are available to aid good visualisation and have been designed specifically to use with, and retract, relevant structures.

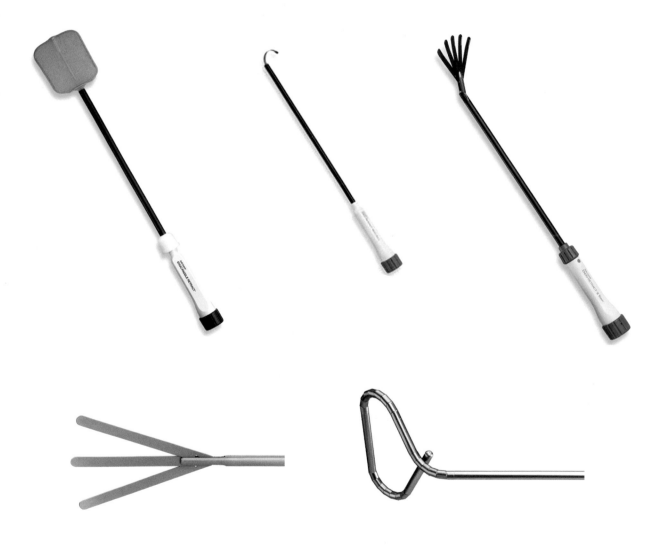

Figure 11.20. Various laparoscopic retractors.

The laparoscopic specimen retrieval pouch

When a specimen or excised structure needs to be removed and is too large to be taken out through the main port incision, a specimen retrieval system can be employed. This allows for the safe removal of structures, such as the gallbladder after a cholecystectomy, without it causing further infection or 'bursting'. This then protects the rest of the abdomen from contamination from its contents. Many of these retrieval pouches are integral within a single-use instrument (■ Figure 11.21). The pouch is contained within the shaft of the introducing instrument and is supported by metallic arms that open once deployed inside the abdomen, keeping it open whilst the specimen is placed inside. The bag can then be closed using an attached string with a slip knot facility to allow it to be removed once the instrument has been removed. It is normally designed to be a one-handed operation, facilitating ease of use.

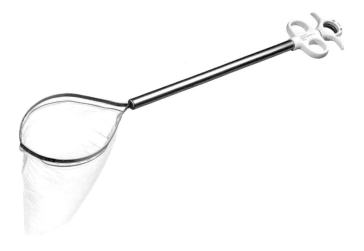

Figure 11.21. Specimen retrieval instrument.

Tissue sealing systems

Various techniques have developed to help the surgeon achieve haemostasis during laparoscopic surgical procedures. Both monopolar and bipolar electrosurgical instruments are used with various applications, from the diathermy hook and monopolar leads attached to dissecting instruments, to specifically designed bipolar instruments. Both have advantages and disadvantages. The 'hook' is used frequently as a dissecting instrument and can be deployed to coagulate small bleeding points as the surgeon dissects. Bipolar instruments are used to coagulate small bleeding vessels that range in size from the smallest to around 3mm in diameter. The main disadvantage to the bipolar instrument is that the jaws become sticky, with a build-up of charred tissue and blood on the jaws of the instrument which inhibits its effectiveness. Thermal spread of the current is wider with bipolar than monopolar instruments, but monopolar produces a greater heat at the tip and can inadvertently cause burns to other surrounding tissue or organs if there is accidental contact with them.

Some coagulators/cutters employ ultrasound technology to seal bleeding vessels whilst used simultaneously to cut through vessels and structures. Bipolar/cutting devices are used in the same way and can seal vessels up to 7mm in diameter. These devices have revolutionised laparoscopic surgery as they can grasp the tissue, seal and transect in one process with the delivery system automatically detecting when optimal cauterisation has been achieved. The harmonic device uses ultrasonic vibrations to cut and cauterise tissue — vibrating at around 55,000 cycles per second, offering greater precision but it takes longer than the bipolar cutter. A selection of bipolar and harmonic tips can be seen in ■ Figure 11.22.

a

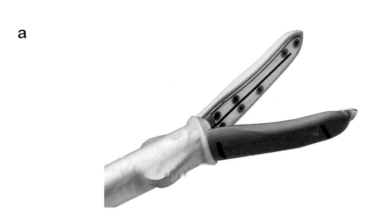

b

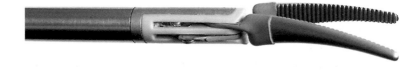

c

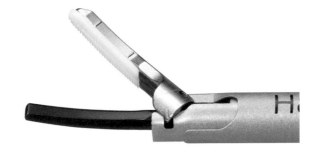

Figure 11.22. a) Bipolar cutter/sealer tip. b) Ordinary bipolar tip. c) Harmonic scalpel.

Laparoscopic stack systems

The development of the camera system and light source, endoinflator, data management system (to record the procedure), and monitors which may be high definition (HD) or 3D, have revolutionised endolaparoscopic surgery. These, when they are all used together, are colloquially known as the 'stack system'. There are many and varied systems available, produced by a number of medical companies but all provide the basic components as described (■ Figure 11.23).

The development of the camera head has revolutionised the surgical view — modern cameras are generally 3-chip full high-definition models which can now be controlled with integrated focus and zoom buttons on the camera head. Monitors are HD and full HD, provided in a range of screen sizes, for example, from 19 inches to 26 inches.

Light sources provide a high brilliance cold light that connects through a light lead to the telescope which has the camera head attached to it. The endoinflator delivers gas into the abdominal cavity (usually carbon dioxide) through a filtered gas inflation tube in one of the entry ports (trocar). The data management system records full patient details, central administration and documentation checklists. It records procedures and captures these as still photographs and video recordings that can be saved by various mediums, DVDs, etc. The procedure can be stored until the data are successfully exported and all patient information is easily accessed to form full reports prior to export.

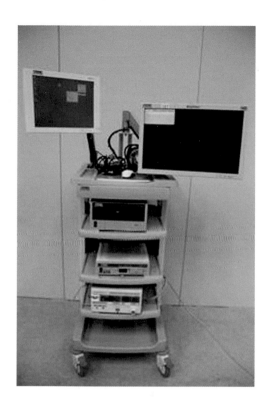

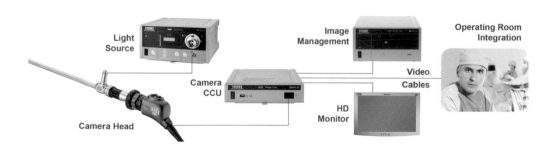

Figure 11.23. A complete stack system on a trolley with an enlarged view of the stack system components. *Image courtesy of Karl Storz.*

Chapter 12

ORTHOPAEDIC INSTRUMENTS AND POWER TOOLS

Orthopaedic surgery is a complex surgical discipline requiring special equipment and instrumentation to meet all the various types of procedures covered within this specialty. The following gives a brief introduction to the continuously progressing developments of this branch of surgery. Some of the instruments that are used in orthopaedics have been mentioned previously, e.g. bone cutters, chisels and gouges (see Chapter 2 — "Instruments for cutting and dissection").

Implants are the most routine aspect of most orthopaedic procedures and include joint prostheses that are many and varied covering hips, knees, shoulders and fingers. Also included are screws, bone plates, rods, intramedullary nails, wires and pins, all requiring specialised instrumentation to facilitate their placement and insertion.

A variety of metal alloys are used in the manufacture of implants; the most frequently used are stainless steel, titanium, cobalt chromium and tantalum. It is important to ensure that implants of the same alloy are used when surgery is performed; if implants of different alloys are placed together, they will corrode and may cause a breakdown or fracture of the implant.

Elevators

Bone elevators are instruments used in most procedures and are found in most orthopaedic sets. They are used to elevate bone and retract tissue from bone so the surgeon can gain access and visualise the operative area, for example, the periosteum needs to be lifted from the bone surface to allow it to be worked on, when repairing a fracture by screw and plate. Examples of a periosteal elevator are the Farabeuf elevator (■ Figure 12.1), the Hohmann elevator (■ Figure 12.2), or the Cobb elevator (■ Figure 12.3). The Cobb elevator is used by spinal surgeons to strip the paraspinous muscle and periosteum off the lamina. Other common elevators include the Bristow (■ Figure 12.4) and Trethowan (■ Figure 12.5) elevators.

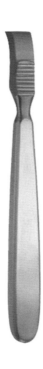

Figure 12.1. Farabeuf periosteal elevator.

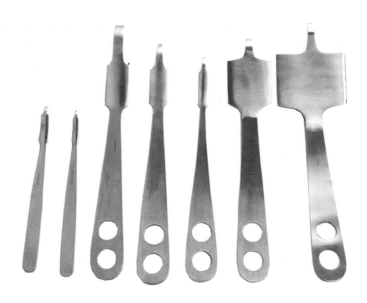

Figure 12.2. Hohmann elevators.

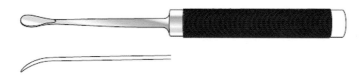

Figure 12.3. Cobb elevator.

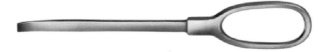

Figure 12.4. Bristow elevator.

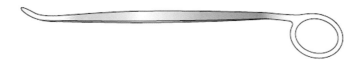

Figure 12.5. Trethowan 'spike' elevator.

Depth gauge

As described under instruments for measuring (Chapter 8 — "Ancillary instrumentation"), the depth gauge (■ Figure 12.6) is used to determine and confirm the depth of a drill hole in bone prior to screw placement so the correct length of screw can be determined.

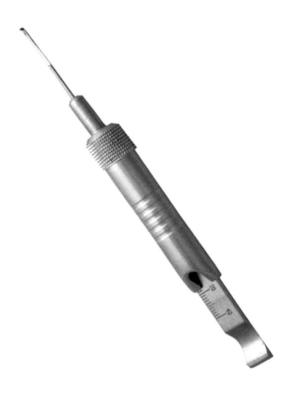

Figure 12.6. Depth gauge.

Screws

The design of orthopaedic screws is varied and may be classified by the following characteristics:

- Conventional screws.
- Locking screws.
- Cannulated screws.

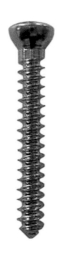

Figure 12.7. Cortical screw.

All have various head configurations and may be self-tapping, non-self-tapping, self-drilling and a combination of both self-tapping and self-drilling. Cortical screws (■ Figure 12.7) have a smaller pitch to the thread and have a greater number of threads along the full length of the screw and are designed to have a strong purchase in the cortical bone. Cancellous screws (■ Figure 12.8) have a greater thread depth, larger pitch to the thread and may be fully or partially threaded. These screws are designed to have a better fixation purchase in cancellous bone.

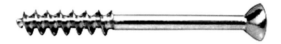

Figure 12.8. Cancellous screw.

The screw driver may have three distinct head slots to fit a particular screw: these may be a star, Phillips (■ Figure 12.9), or hexagonal, the latter being known as AO. The AO system, or Arbeitsgemeinschaft für Osteosynthesefragen (Association for the Study of Internal Fixation) was developed in Switzerland in 1958. Some have a screw-retaining device to hold the screw onto the driver prior to placement (■ Figure 12.10)

Screws can be used to attach implants and plates to bone, or by fixing bone to bone direct. They can also be used to anchor or fix soft tissue.

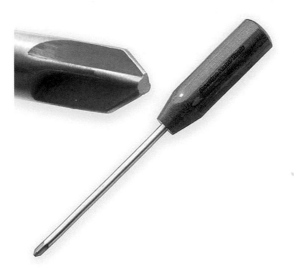

Figure 12.9. Screwdriver showing a Phillips head.

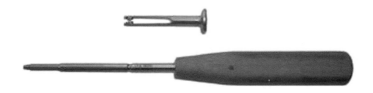

Figure 12.10. Screwdriver showing an attachment to hold a screw in place prior to placement.

Bone-holding forceps

A wide variety of instruments are available to hold bone to facilitate a particular procedure, for example, fixation and holding fractured bone edges in approximation whilst fitting a bone plate to repair the fracture. They may be toothed with serrated edges or just with toothed tips; both with non-locking and locking handles. Some have open jaws so a drill and tap can be placed centrally through the jaws whilst they hold bone fragments together, making them useful for screw placement in plating or lag screwing. Examples of common bone holders are the Lane or Kern (■ Figure 12.11) bone holders (these come with and without locking devices) and the Ferguson bone holder (■ Figure 12.12)

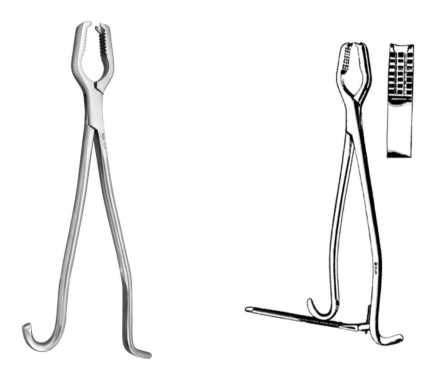

Figure 12.11. Lane bone holder with and without a locking handle.

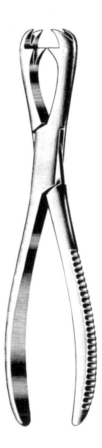

Figure 12.12. Ferguson bone holder.

Mallets

The mallet (■ Figure 12.13) comes in varying sizes depending on the impact required for its use. They are used normally with bone chisels, gouges and osteotomes to cut, dissect and pare bone as described earlier under osteotomes (see Chapter 2 — "Instruments for cutting and dissection").

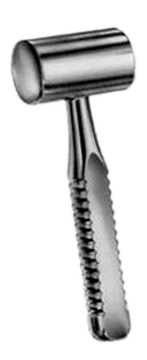

Figure 12.13. Mallet.

Rongeurs

A common surgical rongeur in orthopaedic use is the Kerrison (■ Figure 12.14) and the Bayer or Jansen rongeur (■ Figure 12.15). This instrument is used to open a hole or window in bone. It has a sharp-edged tip which when closed around a plate of bone excises a scoop-shaped piece. The size depends upon the tip being used. Common areas of use are in maxillofacial surgery and neurosurgery where opening a window in the skull is made to gain access to, or expose, the underlying tissue. It can also be used to excise small pieces of soft tissue.

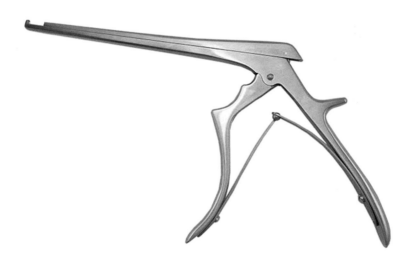

Figure 12.14. Kerrison rongeur.

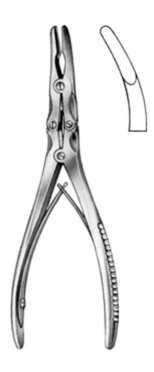

Figure 12.15. Bayer bone rongeur (nibbler).

Bone cutters

Bone cutting forceps are a highly versatile instrument, suitable for a wide variety of orthopaedic procedures. The instrument is available as a straight, direct cutting pair of forceps or with double-action jaws to allow a more comfortable fit around bone. They are available as either straight or angled, and curved on the flat or side. Examples of common bone cutters are the Liston (■ Figure 12.16), Horsley (■ Figure 12.17) or McIndoe (■ Figure 12.18) bone cutters. Single-action cutting forceps are commonly used for cutting smaller bones, where the compound, double-action cutting forceps are used more on larger bones.

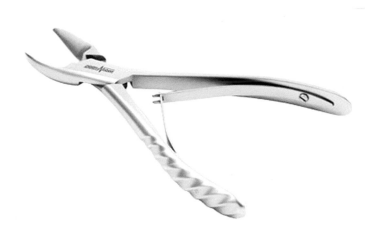

Figure 12.16. Liston bone cutter.

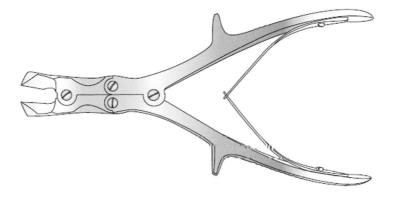

Figure 12.17. Horsley compound-action bone cutter.

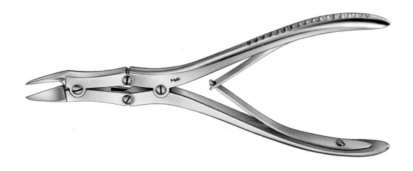

Figure 12.18. McIndoe bone cutting forceps.

Bone rasp

A bone rasp is used in a wide variety of orthopaedic procedures where sculpturing or shaping of bone is required. It is used to smooth rough edges of cut bone and to ream, or clean out hollow bones prior to inserting an implant. The rasp is provided as a single- or double-ended instrument and is shaped with a curved surface allowing an anatomical fit when being used. It is also provided as, and called, a reamer, which is more recognisable as the instrument used prior to the insertion of an implant. The examples below show the different rasps and reamers (■ Figure 12.19).

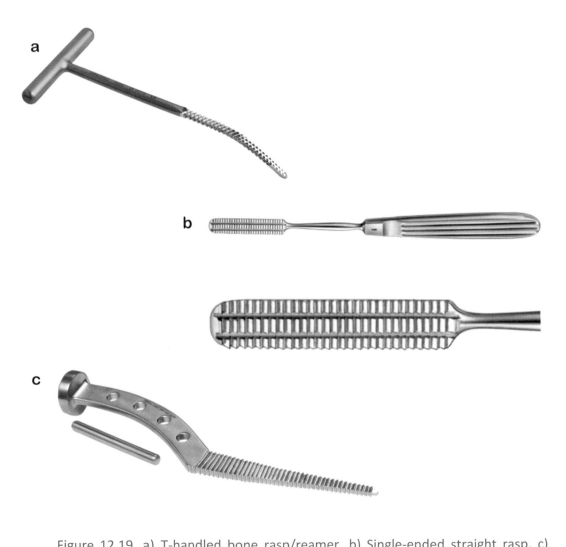

Figure 12.19. a) T-handled bone rasp/reamer. b) Single-ended straight rasp. c) Intramedullary rasp/reamer.

Bone curette

The bone curette is an instrument used frequently in orthopaedic surgery as well as within other specialties. It is a debulking instrument that is used to scrape away tissue and bone from spine, bone and joints. Available in various sizes with different designs of tip curvatures and styles to suite the operative site and procedure, some are double-ended, whilst others are single-ended. A common double-ended curette is the Volkmann curette or 'spoon' (see Chapter 8 — "Ancillary instrumentation") and a single-ended example is the Bruns bone curette (■ Figure 12.20), which has a hollow metal handle allowing a good hold, for the surgeon to exert appropriate pressure whilst in use.

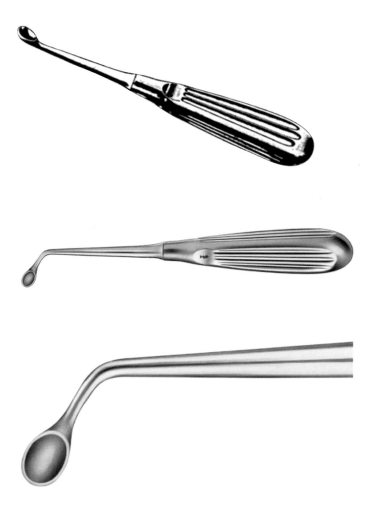

Figure 12.20. Bruns single-ended curette — showing the straight and offset ends.

Surgical wires and pins

Bones are not just held together by plate implants and screws. In many procedures the surgeon uses pins and wires to approximate and hold in place bone fragments and edges together. Kirschner wires, commonly known as K-wires (■ Figure 12.21), are a stainless steel, smooth pin with a sharpened tip and are commonly used in orthopaedics. They come in differing sizes and are used to hold fragments of bone together, being driven into bone by either a power or hand drill. They are commonly passed through the skin into bone, therefore minimising the need for incisions in what may already be a traumatised limb, so reducing the ingress of potential infection. These pins are then removed once bone healing has taken place.

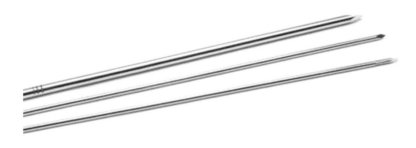

Figure 12.21. Kirschner wires.

Further examples of bone pins are the Steinmann and Denham pins (■ Figure 12.22), which are greater in their diameter than the K-wires and are used where limb traction is the preferred option for fracture treatment using weighted traction on the limb; they are usually used for fractured femurs. The Denham pin is identical to the Steinmann pin except that it has a central short screw thread in the centre of the pin, which when screwed into the cortex of the bone, helps to reduce the risk of the pin sliding through the bone. Both are inserted in the same way, normally with a T-handled chuck or power drill. A Steinmann pin showing both the pointed and triangular ends is shown in ■ Figure 12.22a. These ends fit into the chuck of the T-

a

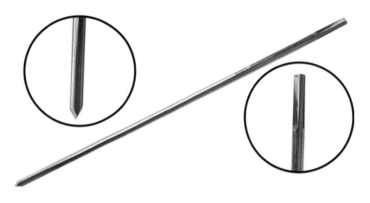

b

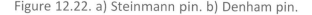

Figure 12.22. a) Steinmann pin. b) Denham pin.

handled insertion instrument (■ Figure 12.23). Both the Steinmann and Denham pins are inserted through the skin and may be placed under general or local anaesthesia.

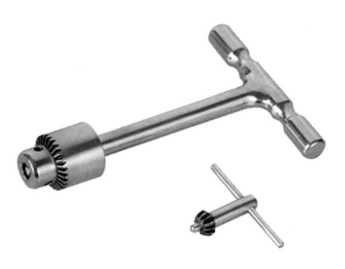

Figure 12.23. T-handle and chuck.

Circulage surgical wire can be used in conjunction with K-wires, putting tension onto a fracture being held by K-wires, or by itself to wrap around bone fragments to hold them in place, approximating bone fragment edges together. The wire is malleable, with enough flexibility to allow shaping and fixation and to be passed around bone using a 'passer' or introducer (■ Figure 12.24).

a

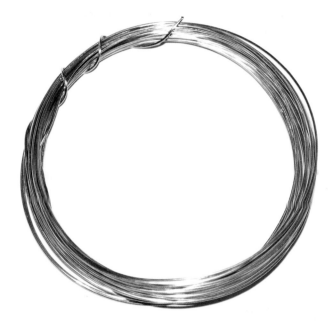

b

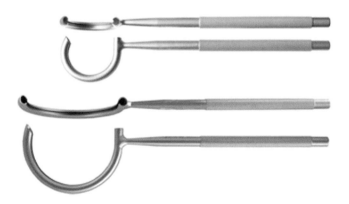

Figure 12.24. a) Circulage wire. b) Wire passer instruments.

There is an obvious need to provide various wire cutters to aid with any wire or pin fixation. ■ Figure 12.25 shows two examples of commonly available wire cutters.

a   **b**

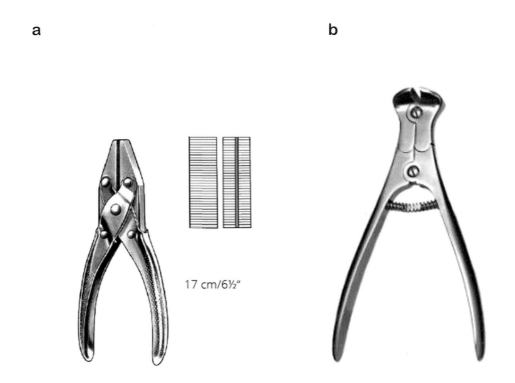

17 cm/6½"

Figure 12.25. a) Pliers. b) Wire cutters.

Power tools

Power tools have now largely replaced the use of hand tools in surgery — mainly in orthopaedics — and have replaced the two main types, namely drills and saws. They provide a key tool in the armamentarium of operating theatre practice within the fields of orthopaedics, neurosurgery, thoracic and dental surgery. These tools have allowed the surgeon to work more efficiently and with more accuracy and have, for the orthopaedic surgeon, revolutionised joint replacement. Orthopaedic surgery is probably more synonymous with the use of power tools and in practice, range in wound management use from drilling, reaming in long bones to the treatment of fractures using screws and nails.

Power tools range in size and have been manufactured for ease of use, as they are lighter in weight, have various power modes of operation and are more consistent in performance. They are powered by battery, compressed air, carbon dioxide and nitrogen gas. The working end (drill bits) and various designs of saw (■ Figure 12.26) are made from metal alloys that are lighter in weight that will generate less

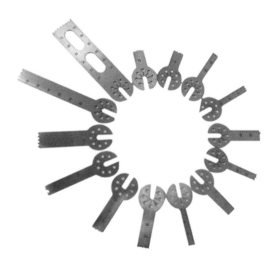

Figure 12.26. A range of saw attachments.

heat when used. They are mainly single use and are disposable devices, so they have an optimum sharpness. The air or gas (pneumatic) operated devices have largely given way to the battery operated devices (■ Figure 12.27), being more ergonomic to use and easier to assemble and operate without a cumbersome cable/lead which can sometimes hinder the manipulation of the instrument.

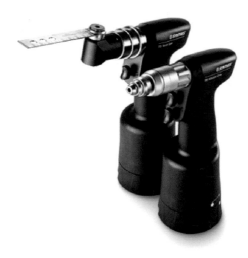

Figure 12.27. Power saw and drill (battery operated).

Larger instruments are used on major bones and joints, while the smaller tools are employed on the smaller bones of the hands and feet, reshaping bone for plastic or reconstructive procedures and to drive pins to stabilise or reduce fragmental fractures.

Power instruments are also used in skin grafting — driving dermatomes and for dermabrasion procedures. Sternal saws are used in cardiac and thoracic surgery and cranial perforator saws are used in neurosurgery.

Most instruments have a wide range of attachments which gives a flexibility of use with drills, saws and reamers. The blades of a saw can be angled in various positions allowing flexible access to cut bone, with coupling and quick change chucks, allowing switching between drills and differing saw blades on the same instrument.

Power saws have either a reciprocating (back-and-forth) action, as with the sternal saw attachment or an oscillating (side-to-side) action, for cutting bone — the blade being available in a variety of sizes and shapes. Drills utilise a rapid rotary motion which can be used to either drill bone for the placement of screws, wires or pins, or if a burr is used (e.g. in dental surgery or for sternal osteotomy) (■ Figure 12.28), they can carve bone. Reamers use a slower rotary motion for reaming the shaft of a long bone to insert intramedullary nails. The speed can normally be altered by the surgeon.

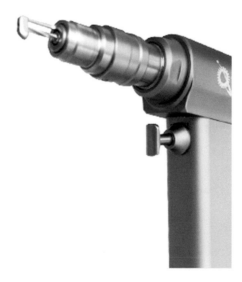

Figure 12.28. Power saw with cranial burr attachment.

Chapter 13

CARDIAC AND THORACIC INSTRUMENTS

Cardiothoracic surgery involves opening the chest through either an intercostal approach or a midline sternal incision (median sternotomy). For cardiac surgery, the chest is opened commonly by an incision along the sternum, of several inches in length. The sternum is then opened using a sternal chisel (■ Figure 13.1), or more commonly a sternal saw.

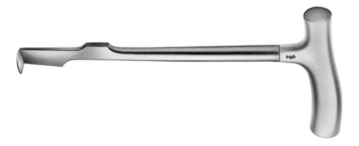

Figure 13.1. Lebsche sternal chisel.

A sternal spreader (■ Figure 13.2) or self-retaining retractor is inserted to open the rib cage to gain access to the mediastinum and heart. Access to the chest for a

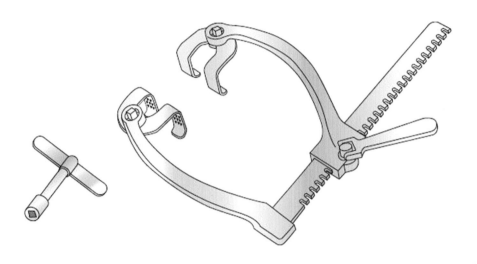

Figure 13.2. Sellor rib spreader.

thoracotomy is usually through a posterolateral approach, through the fifth intercostal space, with the excision of the rib using a rib elevator and rib shears (■ Figure 13.3). A rib spreader is then placed to open the space to gain access to the lung and operative area. For closure of the ribs, an approximator (■ Figure 13.4) is used to bring the ribs back into alignment.

For cardiac surgery, the patient is normally placed on cardiopulmonary bypass which requires specialist cannulas to be inserted (■ Figure 13.5).

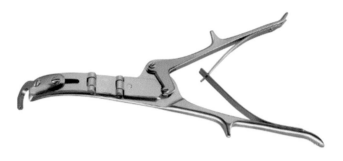

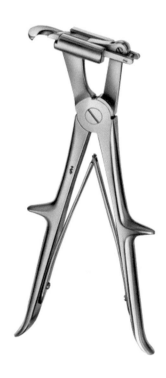

Figure 13.3. Rib shears.

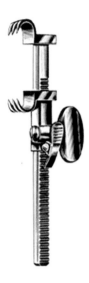

Figure 13.4. Bailey rib approximators.

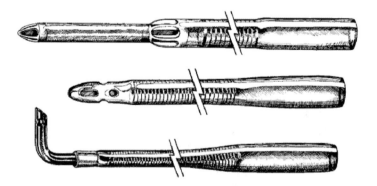

Figure 13.5. Venous cannulas: two-stage (top), cannula for atrial or caval cannulation (middle) and right-angled cannula for paediatric cases (bottom), inserted into the caval-right atrial junction.

Entry into the chest is not possible without the use of rib retractors, rib shears and rib raspatories/elevators. A rib elevator is used to strip the periosteum from the rib before cutting, and both right and left raspatories should be made available; examples of rib elevators are the Doyen and Matson rib elevators (■ Figure 13.6). Other instruments that have specifically been designed for use within these procedures vary

a   b

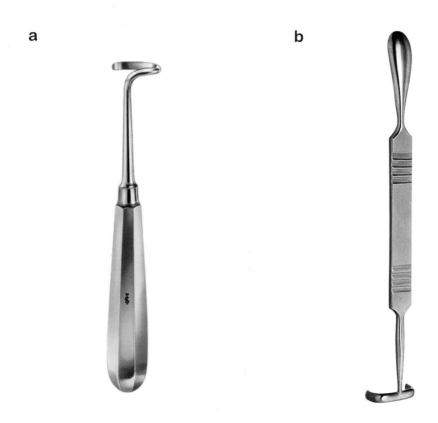

Figure 13.6. a) Doyen rib elevator. b) Matson rib elevator and stripper.

widely and this is dependent upon the procedure being performed. They include bronchus clamps (■ Figure 13.7), rib approximators (■ Figure 13.8) and lung forceps (■ Figure 13.9).

a

b

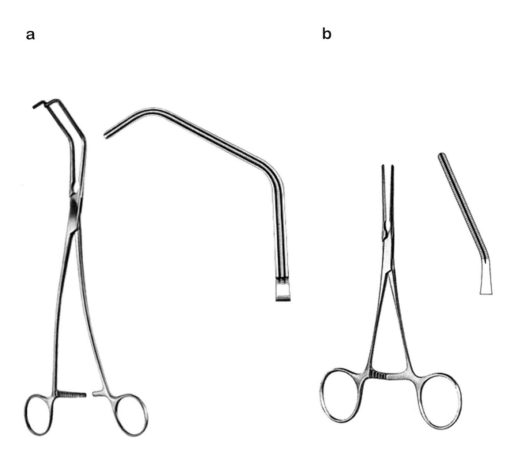

Figure 13.7. a) Bronchus clamp. b) Cooley atraumatic clamp.

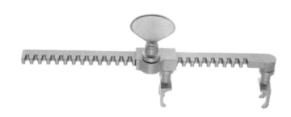

Figure 13.0. Sellor rib approximator.

a   b

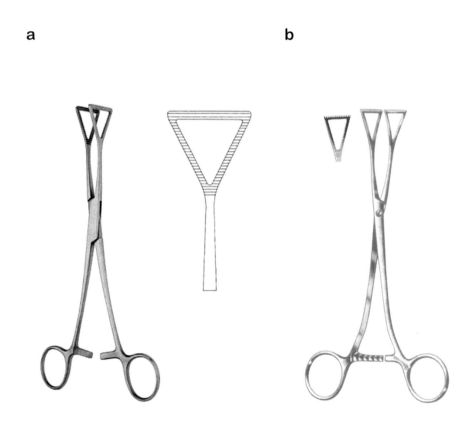

Figure 13.9. a) Lovelace lung tissue forceps. b) Duval lung tissue forceps.

a

b

c

d

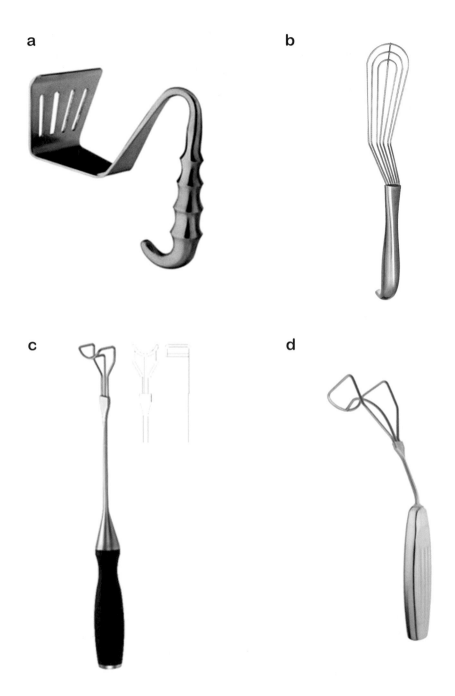

Figure 13.10. a) Davidson scapula retractor. b) Lung retractor/spatula. c) Aortic valve retractor. d) Cooley mitral valve atrial retractor.

Lung and specialist retractors/spatulas also need to be available; these include heart and heart valve retractors (■ Figure 13.10). As mentioned earlier, specialist sternal saws are, in modern practice, usually power saws (■ Figure 13.11). These are, as in orthopaedic surgery, either reciprocating or oscillatory and now more commonly are battery operated.

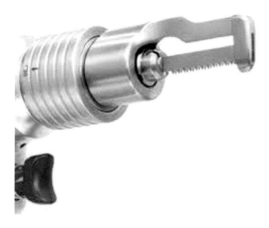

Figure 13.11. Sternal power saw attachment.

Care must be taken when performing a sternotomy as serious damage may occur to underlying structures such as the innominate artery or vein, ascending aorta and pleura. Other instruments that may be used to perform a sternotomy may include sternal shears (■ Figure 13.12), or a Gigli wire saw (■ Figure 13.13).

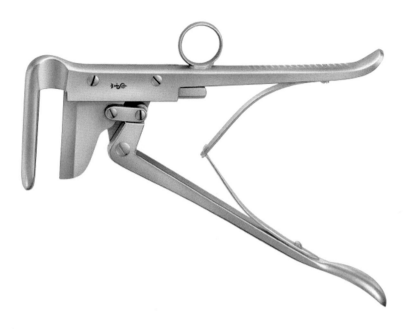

Figure 13.12. Schumacher sternal shears.

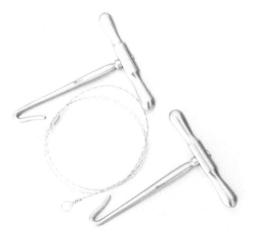

Figure 13.13. Gigli saw with handles.

Chapter 14

THE INSTRUMENT TRAY AND INSTRUMENT SETS

Instruments are assembled into sets or 'trays' for specific specialties or procedures, making it easier for the theatre team, specifically the scrub practitioner, to prepare the correct instruments for any given operating list. The Edinburgh tray system, devised in the 1960s, is a system that is designed to provide a surgical tray layout to make the location of instruments within a particular set functional and safer. It involves the grouping, accessibility and accountability of instruments to be more logical, allowing the scrub practitioner to provide the correct instruments to the surgeon whilst following the procedure; it also provides an easier and more coherent approach to cope with contingencies that may occur during the procedure. The layout of the instruments also allows for a more cogent approach to the instrument accountability when the instrument counts are required at the appropriate times during the procedure. The original Edinburgh tray system included all the 'soft' contents such as the swabs, packs and autoclavable sutures, which were sterilised together with the instruments. It was also deemed appropriate to wrap the trays of instruments in a large enough cover that when opened, it covered the whole trolley top making the set-up process much easier. With the development of more modern and disposable materials used now, this is still very much the same process used today. However, most of the 'soft' materials are pre-packed separately, as are sutures, which are opened as 'extras'.

Depending upon the region, operating theatre or institution, some sets may differ (e.g. a laparotomy set versus a major abdominal set). Most sets are populated by instruments required by the relevant surgeon who dictates the type and number he/she requires. Some procedures require smaller or secondary sets of specialised instruments added to a main or larger, primary set. For example, a major laparotomy set is used to 'open an abdomen' but would need additional instruments to perform specific surgical procedures, such as biliary instruments for a cholecystectomy, or gastric/intestinal instruments for a bowel resection. Other more specialised instruments are available to open separately as single pre-packed instruments.

Ophthalmic sets

These are instrument sets for micro procedures such as cataract removal, or open sets for surgery on eyelids, conjunctiva, rectus muscle, globe and orbit, and retinal surgery for detachment where scleral access is required. Some diagnostic instrumentation may also be required such as lenses for gonioscopy/direct retinoscopy.

Ear, nose and throat sets

These procedures require sets for external ear surgery, e.g. pinnaplasty, plus middle and inner ear surgery. Micro instrumentation is required for procedures with operative access gained through the external auditory meatus such as a myringotomy or tympanoplasty. Nasal procedures such as a submucous resection, rhinoplasty and septal reconstruction require appropriate instruments which may include endoscopic instruments, telescopes and camera stack systems. Sets specific for throat operations include instruments for a tonsillectomy and/or adenoidectomy, as well as open, external throat surgery, e.g. tracheal procedures and thyroid procedures.

Plastic sets

For most basic plastic procedures, a minor instrument set is required with the addition of delicate skin instruments, such as skin hooks and fine scissors. Larger soft tissue instruments are required for procedures such as a mastectomy and breast augmentation/reconstruction. There may also be some small bone instruments for nasal reconstruction (a cross-over with ENT sets). A minor orthopaedic or hand set is required for plastic reconstruction of the hand together with some micro instrumentation for fine reconstruction of nerves and blood vessels (although this might be a combined approach with a vascular surgeon).

Genitourinary sets

The required sets for this specialty can be split between open and endoscopic. The sets for endoscopic procedures include all performed transurethral procedures within the urinary bladder and upper urinary system, cystoscopy, resection of the prostate, bladder tumours and ureteroscopy. When an endoscopic resection is performed, a method of extracting the resected tissue is required which requires the addition of an evacuator to the instrument set, e.g. an Ellik evacuator (■ Figure 14.1).

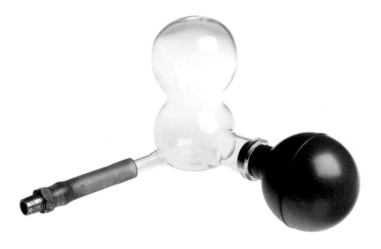

Figure 14.1. Ellik evacuator.

Open procedures require general or minor sets of instruments for most procedures. These cover circumcisions, hydrocoeles, frenuloplasy, for example. Additional instruments need to be added for specific operations such as a vasectomy. Many centres also have special sets available for procedures such as a ureteroplasty and pyeloplasty. For kidney procedures, a major laparotomy set is required with additional vascular and thoracic instruments (a thoracotomy set). Open prostate surgery requires a major abdominal set with long instruments, and Millin and Denis-Browne retractors (■ Figure 14.2).

a   **b**

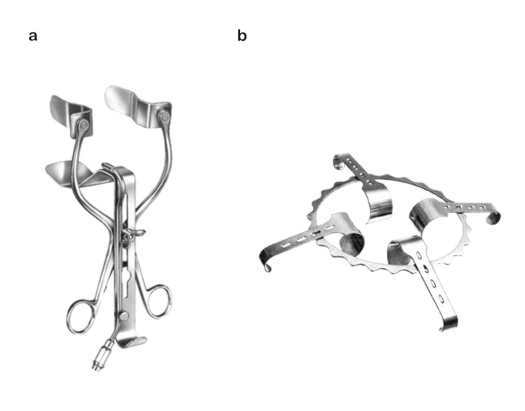

Figure 14.2. a) Millin retractor. b) Denis-Browne retractor.

Orthopaedic sets

Orthopaedic procedures require a general or large bone set which contains soft tissue and basic bone instrumentation. Sets for exposure, reduction and fixation of a bone are required, both for large bones (femur, tibia and humerus, for example) and smaller bones (hand, wrist and feet). These smaller sets may be called small fragment sets and contain smaller instruments to facilitate access to the smaller bones in the hand and feet. Joint replacement requires a specific set that is designed to fit the type of prosthesis being implanted, which includes the necessary reamers and alignment instrumentation/jigs and a large soft tissue set.

Cardiac sets

Cardiac surgical procedures typically require a set of instruments for exposure of the heart and great vessels, and cannulisation for cardiopulmonary bypass. For coronary artery bypass surgery, a separate set is required for saphenous vein harvest or internal mammary artery dissection and anastomosis. The anastomosis of the coronary arteries requires vascular instrument sets which include delicate instruments for dissection and suturing which are normally kept in a separate set. A sternal saw and sternal spreader are required and are packed separately along with internal mammary artery retractors, valve retractors and sizers with aortic and mitral valve dilators for valve replacement.

Thoracic sets

The instruments required for thoracic procedures need to fit the specific thoracic procedure. The main requirements that need to be added to a general set, or included within a specific thoracic set, are instruments needed to remove a rib, e.g. Tudor-Edwards (■ Figure 14.3) or Sauerbruch rib shears. A rib stripper and elevator are also required to be used alongside the rib shears, e.g. the Matson or Doyen rib stripper/elevator (see Chapter 13 — "Cardiac and thoracic instruments"). If thoracic exposure requires a median sternotomy, then a sternal saw and retractor are required in addition. The thoracic set should also have general vascular instrumentation available within or as a separate set. Thoracoscopy is a frequently performed procedure and this requires a separate endoscopic set, with a relevant 'stack system'.

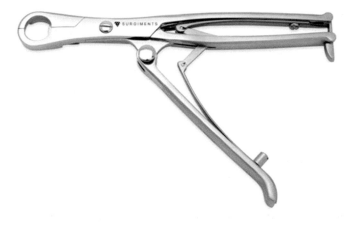

Figure 14.3. Tudor-Edwards rib shears.

Vascular sets

The vascular set is made up of instruments that are required to fit the procedure and are sized accordingly for the exposure, repair, resection and anastomosis of the vessels involved. A laparotomy set or major abdominal set with large abdominal self-retaining retractors is required for the repair of an abdominal aortic aneurysm along with a full range of appropriate arterial clamps both large and small. A general set of instruments with added vascular clamps is sufficient for procedures such as a femoropopliteal bypass or endarterectomy. Peripheral vascular sets are used for carotid surgery, e.g. carotid endarterectomy or the formation of an arteriovenous fistula. Both cardiac and vascular surgery have many common instrumentation requirements.

Gynaecological and obstetric sets

Surgery for obstetrics and gynaecology is very specialised, requiring instruments befitting the needs of the surgeon within these two separate surgical disciplines.

Gynaecological sets of instruments are designed to be used within the field of surgery on adult females — mainly focused on postmenstrual women. Gynaecologists mainly concentrate on the female reproductive system and problems associated with this area, not including pregnancy. Obstetricians focus mainly on the issues surrounding pregnancy and fertility. The instrument sets include instruments for open abdominal, laparoscopic and vaginal surgery. They may have a 'mix and match' approach as some procedures are combined, such as a laparoscopic-assisted vaginal hysterectomy or a total laparoscopic hysterectomy — both of which need access to the cervix through the vagina; for example, with the insertion of a Spackman cannula (see Chapter 10 — "Gynaecological instruments"), which may be required for uterine manipulation. An abdominal hysterectomy is approached via a laparotomy (usually a lower midline incision or a Pfannenstiel incision made below the line of the pubic hair, colloquially known as a 'bikini line' incision). The Pfannenstiel incision is also a commonly used incision for a Caesarean section in obstetrics. The instrument set for a Caesarean is the same as for an abdominal hysterectomy; these are based around the general surgical instruments with additional specialised instruments. Instrument sets are required for dilatation and curettage which provides a basic set for most procedures. These specialist instruments are discussed further in Chapter 10 — "Gynaecological instruments". For obstetric procedures, various forceps are required to aid child birth and vaginal deliveries — these are very specific to obstetric use and can be seen in ■ Figure 14.4.

a

b

c

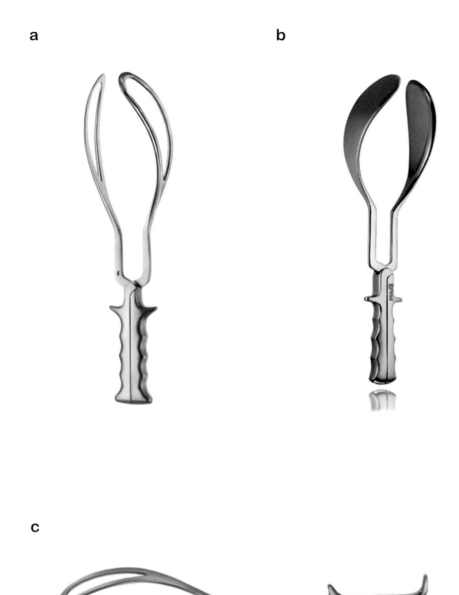

Figure 14.4. Obstetric delivery forceps: a) Simpson-Braun forceps; b) Simpson-Luikart forceps; c) Kielland forceps.

Neurosurgical sets

These instrument sets require specialised microsurgical instruments for surgical procedures on the brain, spinal cord and some peripheral nerves. There may be some cross-over with orthopaedic surgeons as these surgeons sometimes specialise in spinal surgery, performing procedures such as a laminectomy and spinal fusion. For this procedure, there is a need to provide an orthopaedic bone set as well as a selection of neurosurgical instruments. Minor soft tissue sets are sometimes required for soft tissue procedures and repairs. Where a spinal/bone fusion is required, orthopaedic instruments need to augment the other neurosurgical instruments. Power saws and drills are required to enter the skull to perform a craniotomy.

For procedures requiring micro-instrumentation, these need to be compatible with microscopic use; therefore, they need to be anti-glare and designed so the operator's hands and fingers do not obstruct the view, thus they are designed with an 'offset' bend in the handle. An example showing micro scissors with an offset handle is shown in ■ Figure 14.5.

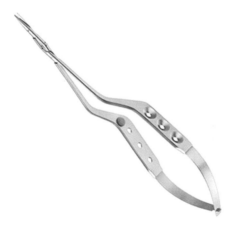

Figure 14.5. Micro scissors with an offset handle.

Laparoscopy instrument sets

These sets (■ Figure 14.6) are mainly made up of general surgical instruments which are normally used to open an abdomen, facilitating an opening required to insert a trocar port, allowing the individual laparoscopic instruments to be inserted. Laparoscopic instruments are described further in Chapter 11. Depending upon the type of laparoscopic surgery being undertaken, this will indicate the type of laparoscopic instruments (and their specific tip designs) to be added and included in the instrument set. These may be from a general surgery, thoracic and gynaecological background and are specific to need. The standard requirements are light leads, a camera, and instruments required to enter the abdomen and to secure a pneumoperitoneum; this may be with the provision of a Veress needle, but always requiring 'gas' tubing to connect to the insufflator.

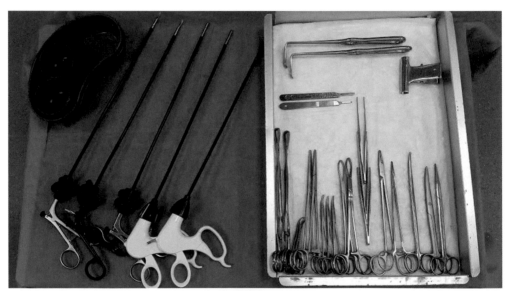

Figure 14.6. A typical laparoscopic instrument set.

The 'general' set

This is the set of instruments (■ Figure 14.7) that can be used for most open procedures and has enough of a variety of instruments to begin the procedure. Further instrumentation or instrument sets can be added as required. For procedures such as open hernia repairs (inguinal, umbilical, ventral, etc.) or an open appendicectomy, this is the set of choice. The choice of instruments within this set, as discussed earlier, may vary between surgeon and institution, but contains the following as a guided example:

- Sponge holders, Rampley.   x 4
- Towel clips.   x 4
- Scalpel handle No.3.   x 1
- Scalpel handle No.4.   x 1
- Dissecting forceps, Lane toothed.   x 1
- Dissecting forceps, Gillies toothed.   x 1
- Dissecting forceps, Adson toothed.   x 1
- Dissecting forceps, DeBakey.   x 1
- Dissecting forceps, McIndoe.   x 1
- Forceps, officer pattern.   x 1
- Scissors, straight, Mayo, 5 inch.   x 1
- Scissors, curved on flat (CoF) 5 inch.   x 1
- Scissors, Metzenbaum, 7 and 9 inch.   x 1 each
- Artery forceps, CoF, Spencer Wells 5 inch.   x 6
- Artery forceps, CoF, Kelly, 7 inch.   x 6
- Artery forceps, Spencer Wells straight, 7 inch.   x 2

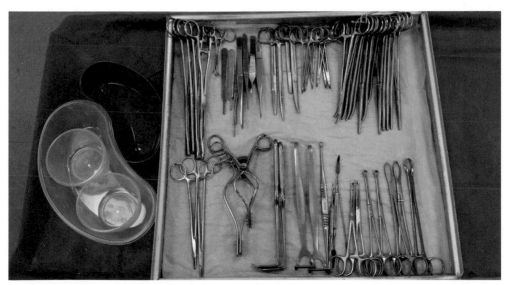

Figure 14.7. A typical 'general' instrument set.

- Artery forceps, Kocher straight.   x 2
- Tissue holding forceps, Babcock.   x 2
- Tissue holding forceps, Allis.   x 2
- Tissue holding forceps, Littlewood.   x 2
- Tissue holding forceps, Lane.   x 2
- Needle holder, DeBakey, 7 inch.   x 1
- Needle holder, Mayo, 7 inch.   x 1
- Retractor self-retaining, Travers.   x 1
- Retractor, Morris.   x 1
- Retractor, Langenbeck.   x 2
- Retractor, Canny-Ryall.   x 2
- Instrument bundle containing:
  - Aneurysm needle;   x 1
  - McDonald dissector;   x 1
  - Volkmann spoon curette;   x 1
  - Sinus probe, 8 inch;   x 1
  - Sinus forceps, Lister 7 inch.   x 1
- Diathermy lead, monopolar.   x 1
- Diathermy forceps, McIndoe, 5 inch.   x 1
- Diathermy quiver and retaining clip.   x 1
- Gallipots, bowls and kidney dish receivers as required.   Normally x 2 of each

Chapter 15

CARE, CLEANING AND STERILISATION

It is of paramount importance to take good care of all surgical instruments, not just for infection control and safety reasons, but also for economic reasons. This equipment is expensive and to replace or repair on a regular basis would be fiscally ruinous to many organisations; it may ultimately reflect on the provision of care and treatment offered to patients within the organisation.

Care of the instruments, in the hands of the scrub practitioner, needs to start with use at the operating table. This, however, is only one aspect of the care required as in reality it starts before, as the instruments and instrument sets are prepared prior to surgery. Once at the operating table, a working partnership with the surgeon and the rest of the theatre team will prevent problems. Good surgical discipline by the scrubbed practitioner, attention to detail by the theatre circulators when opening instruments and sets, and careful handling during the procedure are all important aspects when it comes to the care afforded to the instruments to avoid damage. This will provide protection from harm to both the patient and the operators.

A consistent approach needs to be adopted between the operating theatre staff and the sterile supplies department to ensure that the entire process is understood from preparing instruments, through to dealing with them at the end of the case. Therefore, a robust 'education' needs to be provided between sterile supplies and the theatre staff, with periodic training and reporting between the two departments. These sessions should include reinforcement about the proper handling techniques of all the instruments. The reporting of an instrument defect after use should be dealt with at this meeting with a report of what has been done, what instruments have either been replaced or sent for repair, and how it has affected any particular set of instruments. The direct reporting of a defect should follow the local policy or procedure highlighting the individual problem with any given instrument.

Care of instruments during surgery

Remember that each specific instrument is designed for a particular purpose and to keep it in good order, it must only be used for that purpose:

- Never cut dressings and gauze with surgical dissecting scissors — use scissors within the set supplied for this purpose. Always try to supply the surgeon and assistant with the appropriate scissors to cut sutures, drains and ancillary equipment; always try and discourage the use of tissue scissors.
- Never use forceps to lever, as pliers or openers, or to grasp other larger items that may damage the jaws.
- Do not put strain on the ratchets or joints of instruments — they may crack or break. A weakness in a joint may not be noticed until it is used for its purpose and fails — this could be disastrous at worse, inconvenient at the least.
- Never use elevators or similar instruments as screwdrivers — a common practice which must be discouraged even when the surgeon may be tense.

Prior to use, the scrubbed practitioner should make every effort to check the instruments in the set they are about to use as follows:

- The jaws of the instrument meet appropriately and the serrations in the jaws 'mesh' together evenly.
- The jaws close onto each other without deviation or without having to force them together.
- Check that instruments with ratchets or closure devices do so properly and do not close unevenly — ensure that when closing on a ratchet, that the jaws are fully approximated when the last ratchet on has been reached.
- The edges, tips, jaws and handles are smooth with no 'snags' or burrs.
- Scissors should close smoothly and that the scissor tips close together fully.
- Instruments with ratchets should be easy to close and open, not stiff (which makes it difficult for the surgeon to manipulate) and hold firmly when closed.

Other steps that can be adopted to further the care of the instruments within your control, to protect the instruments within the set during the procedure are outlined below:

- Handle all instruments gently, avoiding weighing them down under heavier equipment and dropping them onto the trolley especially onto their tips (in particular micro instruments). If they are provided in a tray designed with instrument slots, or protective tray inserts, when the instrument is received back onto the trolley, from the surgeon, they should be returned to their respective slot in the tray (■ Figure 15.1).
- Keep instruments within the tray in a coherent order and replace in the tray within this order — this helps with both ease of handling and accountability for the relevant instrument counts.
- Blood, fat and tissue soil should be wiped off the instrument at regular intervals to avoid these drying onto the instrument which hinders its use. This can be achieved by using a dampened swab or by washing in a bowl of sterile water. Prolonged exposure to dried blood can result in corrosion and pitting/rusting of the instrument.

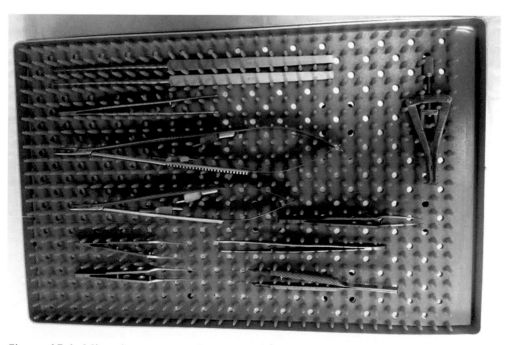

Figure 15.1. Micro instruments in a tray with protective inserts.

All of the above may be described as good "surgical discipline", and should be the aim and watch word of every scrubbed practitioner to avoid both instrument damage and compromised safety.

Instrument counts form an important aspect of instrument care. It is essential not only for patient safety (the inadvertent retention of instruments within a patient) but also to avoid rough handling and instruments being sent with the laundry or thrown in the waste when clearing up after a case. To avoid this, a tracking sheet is included in every instrument set so they may be 'checked in' when preparing for a procedure and 'checked out' after the case has finished — this should avoid any instruments being mislaid or lost. Many instruments may be damaged or broken before they reach the operating theatre if the sets are carelessly packed or handled once they come out of the autoclave. Try to keep the sets in appropriate sized trays and packed without cramming too many instruments into the tray. Handle the tray carefully after sterilisation and do not drop or tip the sets as the instruments may move and get damaged if they fall against each other.

Fundamentals of cleaning

Once the instruments have left the theatre and have been transported back to the sterile supplies department, they should be sent to the receipt area where the instruments are immediately rinsed under warm water to remove all blood, body fluids and tissue. The cleaning cycle is then undertaken in a solution of neutral detergent (pH7).

Most detergents used in the cleaning of instruments are based on an enzymatic cleaning chemical make-up. They are designed for, and are capable of, removing, dislodging and dispersing all forms of soil from the surface of the instrument.

Micro, lumened and delicate instruments are usually processed in an ultrasonic cleaner for a determined time cycle. All instruments should be positioned open with all blades and joints exposed to the cleaning solution, making sure that sharp edges (scissors, etc.) are not touching other instruments. The effects of ultrasonic cleaning are based on the production of sonic waves within the bath that generate minute, micro bubbles on the surface of the item being cleaned. The bubbles then become unstable by expansion, collapse and implode; this generates a localised vacuum which dislodges any soil within or on the instrument. This makes it useful to remove soil from lumened instruments or micro instruments with small parts difficult to get to with conventional hand cleaning.

Some delicate instruments do, however, need manual cleaning, although most are now processed by an automated system (as are the larger instruments), so the important aspect is to pack and place instruments appropriately in the washer trays to avoid damage. Instruments that have an integrated tungsten carbide insert (such as scissors and forceps) should NOT be cleaned with solutions containing benzyl ammonium chloride as this would destroy the tungsten carbide.

After cleaning, the instruments are dried and stored in a clean environment, where they need to be lubricated, if appropriate and needed. The instruments are then placed in their respective sets, checked off against the tracking sheet, and are made ready for sterilisation.

Some instruments can be disinfected only. It is important to be completely aware of the difference between cleaning, decontamination, sterilisation and disinfection:

- Cleaning — is the removal of all bio-burden or soil from the instrument or object's surface.
- Decontamination — is the removal of all pathogenic microorganisms from the instrument to ensure safety when handling them.
- Sterilisation — is the total destruction of all microbiol life including all viruses and spores.
- Disinfection — is the destruction of all vegetative microbiol life, but not spores.

Sterilisation

Most metal devices and instruments are made of materials that are heat stable and therefore are able to undergo sterilisation processes that involve heat and primarily steam sterilisation (under pressure). There has, however, been an increase in device and instrument manufacture that are made of other materials that would be destroyed or damaged by heat (e.g. plastics). These require low temperature sterilisation to avoid damage to components or component parts. Ethylene oxide gas has been used since the 1950s for heat- and steam-sensitive equipment and devices. Other developments have included hydrogen peroxide gas plasma, ozone, peracetic acid immersion and low-temperature steam formaldehyde sterilisers. A basic understanding of these methods of sterilisation is warranted to ensure that instrument and device care is paramount in the back of the scrub practitioner's mind when using such equipment.

To ensure best possible patient care, the care, cleaning and sterilisation of medical devices and instruments that are in contact with sterile body tissues or systems are considered critical within these areas of practice, as any deviation from this critical practice will result in disease or infection transmission.

Before sterilisation of any instrument takes place, the bio-burden of organic matter needs to be fully eradicated; this can only be guaranteed if appropriate and careful cleaning has taken place first. This cleaning of the instruments, whether it is facilitated manually or by an automated system, is the first step to instrument preparation. Various cleaning agents/detergents are used to remove this bio-burden which reduces the number of micro-organisms as well as cleaning off fats, oils, blood and grease. After cleaning (and during, as mechanical washers also perform this), the instruments are disinfected prior to packing for sterilisation.

This section has given a brief overview of the care, cleaning and sterilisation process involved for surgical instrumentation. In reality, this is a much larger topic with much more information, direction and knowledge required for the full and comprehensive understanding of these processes. The reader should read further into this topic and also be guided by manufacturers' guidelines for specific care, cleaning, disinfection and sterilisation. Sterile services is a department that needs to work in close proximity with the operating theatre department — collaboration is key to good practice and ultimately for the care of our patients.

Index